"The primary determinants of disease are mainly economic and social, and therefore its remedies must also be economic and social."

Professor Geoffrey Rose

From *The Strategy of Preventive Medicine* by Geoffrey Rose.
Oxford University Press, 1992.

Acknowledgements

This report is the result of a National Heart Forum initiative which began with an expert meeting on *Social Variations in Coronary Heart Disease: Possibilities for Action*, held in conjunction with the International Centre for Health and Society in 1994. The Forum would like to thank all those who helped with this initiative. Particular thanks are due to:

- The Steering Group for the expert meeting:
  Professor Desmond Julian, National Heart Forum (Chair)
  Ms Mary Cayzer, Community Practitioners' and Health Visitors' Association
  Professor Michael Marmot, International Centre for Health and Society,
    University College London
  Professor Jerry Morris, London School of Hygiene and Tropical Medicine
  Dr Lesley Rogers, National Heart Forum
  Ms Imogen Sharp, National Heart Forum
  Ms Sarah Veale, Trades Union Congress
  Ms Margaret Whitehead, Independent consultant
  Professor Richard Wilkinson, Trafford Centre for Medical Research,
    University of Sussex

- The expert meeting Chairs:
  Sir Douglas Black, Emeritus Professor of Medicine, University of
    Manchester, and formerly President of the Royal College of Physicians
  Professor Jerry Morris, London School of Hygiene and Tropical Medicine

- All the speakers who contributed papers, and all the other participants who contributed to the success of the expert meeting

- The British Heart Foundation for funding assistance for the expert meeting

- Mr Adrian Field, Dr Rosemary Hunt, Ms Henrietta Lang, Ms Rosie Leyden, Mr Chris Wyborn, Ms Tuesday Udell and Ms Jacquie Allix for their contributions to and editorial work on the report.

Social inequalities in coronary heart disease

Opportunities for action

Editor: Imogen Sharp

National Heart Forum
Tavistock House South
Tavistock Square
London WC1H 9LG

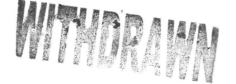

London: The Stationery Office

ISBN 0 11 322105 3

National Heart Forum
Tavistock House South
Tavistock Square
London WC1H 9LG

Registered Company Number: 2487644
Registered Charity Number: 803286
VAT Number: 564 6088 18

Other publications by the National Heart Forum:

At Least Five a Day: Strategies to Increase Vegetable and Fruit Consumption
Coronary Heart Disease Prevention in Undergraduate Medical Education
Coronary Heart Disease Prevention: A Catalogue of Key Resources
Coronary Heart Disease Prevention: Action in the UK 1984–1987
Coronary Heart Disease: Are Women Special?
Directory of Members
Eat Your Words: Healthy Eating and Food Messages
Food for Children: Influencing Choice and Investing in Health
Physical Activity: An Agenda for Action
Preventing Coronary Heart Disease in Primary Care: The Way Forward
Preventing Coronary Heart Disease: The Role of Antioxidants, Vegetables and Fruit
School Meals Assessment Pack

Photographic Credit: cover image:
© Cities Revealed® copyright by the
Geoinformation® Group

Printed in the United Kingdom for The Stationery Office
by Commercial Colour Press Plc, London E7.
J63204 C12 10/98

National Heart Forum

The National Heart Forum (formerly the National Forum for Coronary Heart Disease Prevention) is an alliance of over 35 national organisations concerned with the prevention of coronary heart disease. Members represent the health services, professional bodies, consumer groups and voluntary organisations.

The mission of the National Heart Forum is to work with and through its members to achieve a reduction in coronary heart disease mortality and morbidity rates throughout the UK. It has four main objectives:

- to keep under review the activities of member organisations and disseminate findings

- to identify areas of consensus, issues of controversy, and needs for action

- to facilitate the coordination of activities between interested organisations

- to make recommendations where appropriate.

Member organisations

ASH (Action on Smoking and Health)
ASH Scotland
Association for Public Health
Association of Facilitators in Primary Care
British Association for Cardiac Rehabilitation
British Cardiac Society
British Dietetic Association
British Heart Foundation
British Medical Association
British Nutrition Foundation
Chartered Institute of Environmental Health
Community Practitioners' and Health Visitors' Association
Consumers' Association
CORDA
Coronary Prevention Group
English Sports Council
Faculty of Public Health Medicine
Family Heart Association
Health Education Authority
Health Promotion Agency for Northern Ireland
Health Promotion Wales
National Association of Governors and Managers
The NHS Confederation

Northern Ireland Chest, Heart and Stroke Association
Royal College of General Practitioners
Royal College of Nursing
Royal College of Paediatrics and Child Health
Royal College of Physicians of Edinburgh
Royal College of Physicians of London
Royal College of Surgeons of England
Royal Institute of Public Health and Hygiene and the Society of Public Health
Royal Pharmaceutical Society of Great Britain
SHARP (Scottish Heart and Arterial disease Risk Prevention)
Society of Cardiothoracic Surgeons
Society of Health Education and Health Promotion Specialists
Society of Occupational Medicine
Trades Union Congress
The Wellcome Trust

Observer organisations

Department of Health
Department of Health and Social Services, Northern Ireland
Medical Research Council
Ministry of Agriculture, Fisheries and Food
National Consumer Council
Scottish Consumer Council
Scottish Office, Department of Health
Welsh Office

In addition, a number of distinguished experts in the field have individual membership.

Contents

Foreword

Coronary heart disease is the leading single cause of death in the UK, killing over 400 people each day, or 150,000 people a year. It causes illness and disability for many more.

Death rates from the disease in the UK have been declining, though at a slower pace than in similar developed countries such as the United States and Australia. However, what is striking is that in the UK the social class differences in coronary heart disease death rates are widening, and the disease has become increasingly associated with disadvantage.

Much of this widening gap is due to the greater reductions in death rates from coronary heart disease among non-manual groups, between the early 1970s and the 1990s. Among social class I men, for example, the death rates have halved. Reductions among manual groups over this period have been much less dramatic and, among social class V men, there has actually been a small increase in coronary mortality. By the early 1990s, coronary mortality among unskilled men of working age was three times that of professional men in the same age group.

The aim of this National Heart Forum initiative is to contribute to an overall reduction in coronary heart disease, by examining the reasons for the social class differences in the disease, and setting out strategies and policy options to reduce these inequalities. This report derives from a National Heart Forum expert meeting in 1994 which brought together over 70 researchers, policy-makers, health and social practitioners, and government representatives. The research presented at the expert meeting has been updated in the light of recent evidence. The report's conclusions also take account of the findings of the National Heart Forum's agenda-setting initiative, *Coronary Heart Disease Prevention: Looking to the Future*.

The fact that the social class inequalities in coronary heart disease have widened means that they can also narrow: the social and economic policies which contributed to them could also be used to raise the standards of the worst to those of the best. As the UK's leading single cause of death, coronary heart disease could be used as a test case for tackling health inequalities. Addressing the wider social factors which contribute to the development of coronary heart disease could also help to reduce the incidence of many other diseases which share some of the same determinants and risk factors.

The challenge is to engage not just health professionals, who have described the problem, but also those social policy-makers and practitioners, in government and beyond, whose work will have a real impact on addressing the root causes. Fresh approaches are needed to tackle not only the social differences in behavioural risk factors, but also the social inequalities inherent in education, welfare, income and work. Tackling these from a young age must be a priority.

With health inequalities once more on the political agenda, and coronary heart disease a national priority, this report should prove both useful and timely. We are grateful to the British Heart Foundation for providing financial assistance for this National Heart Forum initiative. We hope that the report will stimulate action to reduce the widening social class differences in illness and death from coronary heart disease across the UK.

Professor Desmond Julian CBE MD FRCP
Chairman, Steering Group
Chairman, National Heart Forum (1993–1998)

Chapter 1

The way forward: summary and recommendations

Coronary heart disease is the leading single cause of death in the UK, killing 150,000 people each year. Although death rates from the disease have fallen since the 1970s, the reductions have been greater among higher socioeconomic groups. In the UK there are now large – and widening – social class gradients in mortality from all cardiovascular diseases (including coronary heart disease and stroke). In the early 1970s, the coronary heart disease mortality rates of unskilled (social class V) men were 25% higher than those of professional men (social class I). By the early 1990s, however, there was a three-fold difference. This has resulted from a small increase in mortality rates in social class V men since the 1970s but a huge reduction – a halving of rates – among professional men. Among women the gap firstly narrowed and then widened again. This socioeconomic gradient is also reflected in morbidity rates, with angina, heart attack (myocardial infarction) and stroke all more common among those in manual social classes. Furthermore, it is not only social class differences in coronary heart disease that are widening; inequalities in risk factors for the disease, such as smoking and aspects of nutrition, are also increasing.

The fact that the social class distribution in coronary heart disease and the size of the gap have changed over time shows that these inequalities are not fixed. If they can get worse, they can also get better. The trends are the result of conscious social and economic policies, so such policies can also be used to reverse them. Furthermore, the differences in the magnitude of social class differences in coronary heart disease between different countries also suggest that there are changeable causes that can and need to be addressed.

The national health strategies in England, Scotland, Northern Ireland and Wales, with a focus on reducing health inequalities, improving the health of the worst off in society, and cross-sector working, provide a useful framework for action.

A national strategy to reduce social inequalities in coronary heart disease

1 A comprehensive national strategy to address social inequalities in coronary heart disease is needed. Such a strategy should aim to reduce overall rates of coronary heart disease by reducing the particularly high rates among disadvantaged social groups. As part of this, national and local targets for reducing social class inequalities in coronary heart disease mortality should be set and monitored.

2 Coronary heart disease should be used as a test case for tackling health inequalities.

Social inequalities in coronary heart disease need to be reduced for several reasons. Firstly, the overall health of the nation cannot be effectively improved without addressing health inequalities. It will be difficult to achieve the targets for reducing coronary heart disease if the health of only half the population is improving. Life expectancy would be improved if all groups in society were becoming healthier. Secondly, there are ethical reasons for concern. Thirdly, the implications of ignoring the social gradient in coronary heart disease include not just costs to the health service, but also human costs and economic costs: human capital and social exclusion are major influences on national prosperity. Coronary heart disease has major consequences for the UK economy, with annual costs of £10,000 million, including £1,600 million in direct health care costs (mainly treatment), and £8,400 million in indirect costs (mainly loss of production, due to both sickness and premature death). Each year, some 65 million working days are lost because of sickness caused by coronary heart disease.

There is already sufficient research describing the existence of health inequalities. There is now a need for action. With the government's focus on reducing health inequalities, and coronary heart disease as a national priority with targets, the time is ripe for a national strategy to reduce inequalities in coronary heart disease. Reducing inequalities in coronary heart disease will also reduce inequalities in other diseases, such as stroke and cancer, whose determinants and risk factors are similar. Coronary heart disease provides a useful focus for tackling the underlying social factors causing ill health, and for measuring specific risk factor and physiological outcomes and should be used as a test case for action to reduce health inequalities.

Tackling the determinants of ill health will require action which cuts across government departments and involves a wide range of agencies at national, international and community levels. Cabinet level commitment is essential, and the national health strategies provide scope for real cross-departmental initiatives and cross-sector involvement. A comprehensive national strategy, with considerable long-term investment, will be needed to make a serious impact on reducing social inequalities in coronary heart disease. Such a strategy should address:

- the underlying social and economic factors that increase general susceptibility to ill health, and the impact of social, economic and health policy on the health and well-being of the population

- the environmental factors that sustain unhealthy behaviour, and

- the individual's behaviour.

Both broad social policy strategies and strategies specific to individual diseases or risk factors are needed to tackle health inequalities. In the past, for example, serious diseases such as tuberculosis, rheumatic fever and syphilis – all strongly linked to social conditions – have been virtually eradicated primarily through a combination of social programmes and social policy measures. Action at international, national and local levels is needed.

A life course approach

3   **The national strategy should adopt a life course approach to reducing inequalities in coronary heart disease, beginning with a focus on children, and addressing general deprivation and susceptibility.**

The social gradient in ill health is apparent for all causes of death apart from breast cancer, indicating that general susceptibility may play a part in causing inequalities in coronary heart disease. Such a general susceptibility is partly biological – possibly nutritional – and is exacerbated by social conditions and economic circumstances: general deprivation is likely to magnify any biological disadvantage.

The interplay between socioeconomic disadvantage and biological susceptibility begins in early life – manifested in high infant mortality, and low birthweight and weight at one year, for example – carries on through childhood and adolescence, and tends to continue throughout a person's life course. Deprivation has an impact at all stages, and a number of factors are important including, for example, maternal and childhood nutrition, prevalence of illness during childhood, educational opportunities and attainment and, in adulthood, working conditions and unemployment, chances of smoking, and social conditions. Eventually, the impact of such deprivation leads to higher morbidity rates, and a greater chance of premature death.

Coronary heart disease is one disease where such an interplay is clearly at work. Thus, strategies for prevention and risk reduction should take a life course approach – beginning before birth, and tackling social and economic disadvantage as well as individual health behaviour. There is increasing evidence that what happens in the womb (foetal development) and in the first year of life are important determinants of coronary heart disease risk in middle age. Furthermore, where past infant mortality rates have been high and thus, by implication, children nutritionally deprived, coronary heart disease mortality rates 70 years later are also high. Cumulative social class is strongly related to cardiovascular risk: a person's *father's* social class as well as *their own* social class seem to be important contributors to cardiovascular mortality, indicating the long-lasting influences of socioeconomic circumstances in childhood on mortality in adulthood.

What is most important, however, is the recognition that the increased coronary risk that disadvantage brings is sustained from birth to adulthood, and that experiences at different stages of the life course have different effects. Furthermore, behaviours that affect later coronary risk are often formed in childhood. For example, eight in ten smokers begin before they reach the age of 20; and those who exercise at a young age are more likely to continue being physically active as they get older. Research also suggests that childhood nutrition has important long-term health consequences.

It is therefore important to start tackling health inequalities at a young age, and to make children and young people a main focus of any strategies to reduce inequalities in coronary heart disease. Reducing unequal exposure to factors detrimental to health throughout the life course demands considerable long-term effort. The Department of Health has concluded that "it is likely that accumulative differential lifetime exposure to health-damaging or health-promoting physical and social environments is the main explanation for observed variations in health and life expectancy."[1] The government's commitment to improve education is welcomed, particularly as the number of years of education, and educational attainment, seem to be important in determining rates of coronary heart disease in later life. However, there is also a need to create a culture of opportunity and optimism throughout the life course, perhaps through the programme of the Social Exclusion Unit.

Need for broad-based interventions

4   **Interventions to reduce inequalities, at national and local levels, should be broad-based, and include a combination of structural or social policy measures and health promotion initiatives.**

Broad-based intervention programmes are needed to address health inequalities. Traditionally, many of the interventions have been small-scale, started at local level in response to a local need. Often too, the resources invested in such interventions have been small and short-term.

Research has shown that interventions to reduce social inequalities in coronary heart disease need to be broad-based and to include a combination of measures. The most successful are those that involve structural or social policy measures as well as health promotion. Health education interventions that provide a combination of information and personal support are also successful. There is evidence that traditional health education, based on mass media or written information, does not necessarily change behaviour in 'hard to reach' groups, and may therefore exacerbate social class differences. Written information alone rarely works, and among lower socioeconomic groups, more personal approaches are far more effective.

Initiatives which are integrated with existing social and health services – rather than 'tacked on' – are more likely to reach the target group and be effective and sustained in the long term. It is therefore important to 'institutionalise' initiatives. Considerable extra investment in terms of both time and money is necessary to reach the 'hard to reach' groups.

Tackling material conditions

The pattern of income distribution within a country seems to have an important effect on health, including mortality rates and life expectancy. Countries with a less equitable income distribution and greater differences in income have higher premature coronary heart disease rates and shorter overall life expectancy. Income distribution therefore seems to explain some of the variations in coronary heart disease mortality rates between countries. Furthermore, changes in income distribution over time also seem to be associated with the rate of decline of mortality rates: countries which experience a reduction in income differences and become more egalitarian also experience a faster rate of decline in coronary heart disease mortality. These patterns are particularly marked, and therefore important, among younger age groups, and among women.

There is now sufficient evidence that income inequalities cause ill health, and action to redress those inequalities is needed at both national and community or local levels. Health inequalities show a continuous social gradient across income groups; there is not a simple cut-off point. Greater health inequalities are also likely to contribute to higher overall mortality rates. Effective policies to tackle them may be one of the best ways of improving national mortality rates.

Two features of income differentials are important. Firstly, income differentials may be an indicator of the overall social environment that affects the health of the whole population. Secondly, the poorer the poor become, the worse their social conditions become and the poorer their health. Since income differentials do not seem to be necessary for economic growth, there does not need to be a trade-off between economic policies and population health.

It seems that income differences within countries amplify differences in social status, and most of the health inequality seems to result from the influence of low relative income on the mortality rates of the relatively poor. It may be that, in less egalitarian societies, this is caused by awareness of social differences, of inferiority or superiority, of failure and social exclusion, of low social status and loss of self-esteem. This would link with research highlighting the importance of psychosocial factors – such as a sense of control, social support and job security – for health and health inequalities, perhaps through a pathway of chronic stress.

In the UK, the increase in health inequalities and the social gradient in coronary heart disease mortality, particularly among men, has been mirrored by widening income differences over the same period. There has been an increase in the absolute numbers of poor families in the UK, and increasing social polarisation. For example, there has been a three-fold increase in lone parenthood since the early 1970s and a doubling of long-term unemployment. By 1998, more than one in three children were living in poverty – compared to less than one in ten in 1979. Overall, income inequality in the UK widened more rapidly during the 1980s than in any other developed market economy and, at the same time, the UK's relative position in the international life expectancy league table slipped.

5   In order to reduce health inequalities, there needs to be cross-government commitment and action at Cabinet level, including integration of social, economic, health and environmental policies. As a priority, health impact assessments should be used to assess the health implications – including the implications for coronary heart disease – of government economic and social policies.

Government economic and social policies are likely to have a greater impact on health than the kinds of factors that health professionals and community workers can change at a local level. In order to tackle social class differences in cardiovascular disease risk, it will be necessary to address the causes of social inequalities, as well as the material basis of social gradients in risk factors such as diet and smoking. To achieve this, the government's social, economic, health and environmental policies need to be fully integrated. In particular, one of the first principles should be that economic policy takes account of the health implications of its effects. Any concerted attempt to tackle social inequalities in coronary heart disease inevitably involves social policies beyond the health system.

Reducing income inequalities, including addressing relative deprivation and material conditions, is likely to be one of the most effective ways to reduce inequalities in coronary heart disease. For example, a person's income influences where and in what type of housing they live, their educational opportunities, and their access to healthy food, transport and leisure facilities, and health care.

However, the solution is not simply to increase cash income or benefits, as this does not address the community-based nature of the problem. A goal must be to restore opportunities and reasons for optimism among the whole of society, including the poor and increasingly socially excluded, and to offer them some means to control their own lives. Once people have a future that they can believe in, they will value their life and want to protect it. The Social Exclusion Unit should address this issue as a priority. Welfare-to-work should be linked to welfare-to-health, as poor health is a barrier to work for many poor families.

Essential elements of a strategy to improve material conditions also include a reconsideration of indirect taxation, which has increased and which penalises the poor, and of benefits such as free school meals. The state benefit system needs to be reviewed, as some people are simply too poor to live and eat healthily. In particular, a review of the food cost element in benefit payments is needed, with the food element ring-fenced at a level which allows a healthy diet.

6   Local health strategies, drawn up under Health Improvement Programmes and Health Action Zones, should focus on reducing health inequalities by reducing social disadvantage and deprivation and improving material conditions. Coronary heart disease could be used as a test case.

In local communities, health is not evenly distributed: those living in more deprived areas also have poorer health and higher premature mortality. The type of neighbourhood is associated with risk factors such as diet, smoking and physical activity, independently of social class and income. It is therefore important to pay attention to the characteristics of local neighbourhoods as well as to individuals living within them.

Local health plans, or health strategies, should focus on reducing inequalities in coronary heart disease by improving material conditions and the quality of life. Such plans, based within Health Improvement Programmes and Health Action Zones, could tackle deprivation, urban regeneration, transport, safety, and community involvement, for example, as well as education and training. They should be led by health authorities and local authorities as part of their public health responsibilities and should be based on four principles: partnership; integration of local economic, social and environmental policies; local participation; and redistributive policies across social groups and across the life cycle. Evaluation of such initiatives is essential.

Partnership: Local partnerships involving a wide range of statutory and non-statutory organisations are needed, to agree and implement the local health plan and policies to improve the community's health. Senior representatives of health and local authorities, business, voluntary groups and academia, for example, should be involved, to provide accountability and commitment to real and sustainable resources.

Integration of local economic, social and environmental policies: As part of the health plan, an integrated investment strategy in deprived areas might cover industrial business development, housing, health care, shopping and leisure facilities, and the environmental infrastructure. It could include:

- opportunities for local employment, and economic incentives aimed at producing more fairly-paid jobs in the community

- local transport policies to enable people to get easily to work, shops, and health and leisure facilities, as well as minimising accidents and enabling safe play and activity

- action plans to address food availability and cost, aimed at retailers, wholesalers and producers, as well as consumers, and

- improvements to housing, including action following social and physical surveys and energy audits, and a reduction in damp and cold housing.

The long-term aim should be to enable people to move into better life circumstances, including well-paid work, as an essential element of a strategy to improve health. Particular attention needs to be given to families receiving housing benefit, clothing grants and free school meals, among whom building optimism will be vital.

Local participation: Local people need to be involved in decisions on local health improvements. Consultation on perceived health needs and on opportunities to improve health is important so that communities are involved in how their money is spent, and participate in the process of building sustainable communities.

Redistributive policies across social groups and across the life cycle: It may be necessary to allocate resources unequally, targeting those most in need, in order to enable all socioeconomic groups to benefit from health promotion measures.

Evaluation: Evaluation of local initiatives will be essential, and will need to include different process and outcome measures. Earmarked funds, to enable evaluation of the effectiveness of local community initiatives, would be useful at both a national and local level.

Behavioural factors

7   **The Department of Health, with other partners, should develop a strategy to tackle the wider determinants of health behaviour, and factors which sustain unhealthy behaviours, with a focus on health lifestyles of children and young people.**

Changing health behaviour has been a traditional focus of health education and health promotion. However, while health lifestyles are important, a large proportion of the social class differences in coronary heart disease both within and between countries remains, so far, unexplained by health behaviour: research internationally has found that adjusting for a wide range of 'traditional' risk factors, including smoking, blood cholesterol levels and blood pressure, does not totally remove the social class differences in cardiovascular disease.

However, widening social class differences in coronary heart disease are also reflected in social gradients in health behaviours, such as smoking and some aspects of nutrition, which tend to follow the contours of deprivation. There is a need to address the factors which sustain these social gradients, and to understand the factors that enable some people in deprived groups to have healthier lifestyles, such as giving up smoking.

Therefore, while it is important to address behavioural factors, this should be only one part of a wider strategy to tackle inequalities in coronary heart disease.

There is evidence that health education strategies which focus on the individual may exacerbate health inequalities, by having most impact on higher social classes. Thus, there is a need for a shift in emphasis away from the individual, to address the wider determinants of health behaviour and the environment in which people live. Healthy choices need to be made not only easy, but also possible. Strategies are needed which tackle the supply-side rather than simply consumer demand, and address social and psychological factors. This might include addressing availability of and access to a healthy diet, as well as providing information on nutrition and cheap sources of important nutrients; and tackling the factors that sustain smoking among low income groups.

The priority needs to be on initiatives which tackle health behaviours among children and young adults, since many health behaviours, such as smoking and physical activity patterns, are established early in life.

Smoking

8   **The government should develop and implement a comprehensive tobacco strategy aimed at reducing smoking rates among disadvantaged groups, and should allocate additional resources to new initiatives.**

Cigarette smoking is a major preventable cause of coronary heart disease, and smoking patterns reflect the social class gradient in the disease. Smoking has become increasingly concentrated among low income groups, particularly those with children. Since the early 1970s, smoking rates have fallen among higher and middle income groups, but have remained unchanged among the bottom income groups, and 27% of smokers are now concentrated in the lowest 10% income group. This pattern is also found among younger ages (thus ruling out any possible bias associated with deaths from smoking-related diseases). Although the proportion of lone parents who smoke has remained at 60%, there are now three times as many lone parents as in the mid-1970s.

Smoking is further concentrated among the most disadvantaged low income families, a pattern that remains invisible to official statistics. For each marker of social disadvantage – social tenancy (living in council or housing association accommodation), having no educational qualifications, and manual work – smoking rates almost double. The important causal factor in continuing to smoke seems to be long-term poverty.

Most poor smokers want to give up, and some succeed. As a first step, it is important to identify what helps poor smokers give up, and the factors that make giving up more likely.

A major plank of national tobacco policy is to raise prices through tax increases. While this has an important effect on reducing overall tobacco consumption, it has not reduced rates among the poorest smokers and additional targeted tobacco strategies, linked with family welfare policies, are needed to help low income smokers give up. As a priority, some of the tobacco tax revenue that low income smokers return to the Treasury should be used to fund new and innovative interventions. A comprehensive and integrated multi-level strategy is needed, and might include the following initiatives:

- Anti-smoking aids, such as nicotine replacement patches and gum, could be made available on prescription through the NHS, making the means to give up smoking free for those who most need it. Targeting could be improved further by making such nicotine replacement therapies available as a 'passported' benefit for those on means-tested social security benefits, alongside help with dental and optical costs. Primary care teams have a particularly important role in reaching deprived groups.

- Community-based, outreach health promotion programmes could back up such initiatives.

- Availability of child-care facilities could be improved, to help reduce smoking among low income mothers. It is important that initiatives also address the psychosocial aspects of smoking. For example, for lone mothers cigarettes often represent 'time out' from children.

- Welfare-to-work policies should be linked with welfare-to-health policies: success in smoking cessation is associated with optimism.

- Smoking among young people should be a priority, as smoking behaviours are formed early in life. Additional resources are needed for smoking education to counter tobacco promotion.

Diet

9   **A national food strategy is needed to improve the diets of the most disadvantaged, particularly by increasing their consumption of vegetables and fruits, and increasing the P:S ratio (the ratio of polyunsaturated fats to saturates). Such a strategy should address cost, availability and access, and food skills, and should tackle the material basis of nutritional inequalities.**

Nutrition is fundamental in the development of coronary heart disease, and is possibly the main cause of 'general susceptibility' among lower income groups. In particular, research suggests that childhood nutrition and maternal diet during pregnancy have important long-term effects on health in later life.

The foods offering the greatest protection against coronary heart disease show the greatest inequalities in consumption. Social class differences are greatest in vegetable and fruit consumption, and in the ratio of polyunsaturated fats to saturated fats (the P:S ratio). In contrast, there is little social class difference in the percentage of energy consumed from fat. These patterns begin early in life. For example, within their first year, infants from manual groups eat 50% less fruit than those in non-manual families. The diets of low income families are also characterised by a lack of variety. Furthermore, the nutrition gap between social groups is widening; for example, the intake of antioxidants (found in vegetables and fruit) among the poorest households has declined over the past two decades.

A national food strategy to improve the diets of the most disadvantaged should focus on increasing vegetable and fruit consumption, and increasing the P:S ratio. It would need to acknowledge the limits that poverty and debt impose, and address the material basis of unhealthy diets. As well as addressing cost, availability and access, and food skills, agencies should also tackle the commercial pressures for foods which promote an unhealthy diet. Practical solutions are available, and need to be implemented.

A national food strategy should include:

- free school meals, including breakfast, at least for children in low income families. The school meals should meet minimum nutritional standards.

- a national school vegetable and fruit scheme, including free fruit and vegetables for children

- an extra dietary allowance for low income women who choose to breastfeed

- the availability of social fund grants, rather than loans, for essential items such as cookers and fridges

- a review of the food cost element in social benefit payments. The food cost element should be made explicit and be ring-fenced at a level which permits a healthy diet.

- a commitment not to levy VAT on food. This would be a regressive tax because the poor spend proportionally more of their income on food.

A healthy and varied diet consistently costs more than a monotonous, unhealthy diet, and many cheap, high calorie foods are also high in fat and sugar. Low income families spend a higher proportion of their income on food, but also tend to be more efficient purchasers of nutrients. Pricing policies, and new ways to make healthier foods cheaper, are needed at both an international and national level, perhaps using subsidies, so that the overall cost of a healthy diet is reduced. Such policies should include:

- reform of the Common Agricultural Policy, and particularly the fruit and vegetables regime, which has a disproportionately greater effect on people on a low income.

- restricting the profit margin levied on food prices by UK retailers. The profit margins achieved by UK retailers are up to four times higher than those in other European countries for example.

Information and education

There are no significant differences between different income groups in levels of knowledge about a healthy diet, or in skills in preparing or cooking food, but education about food and nutrition is inadequate for all groups. It is important that the information environment supports healthy eating advice, and that the commercial pressures on consumers to buy foods high in fat, sugar and salt are addressed.

- Codes of practice governing the commercial advertising of foods to children, including TV advertising, need to be tightened. Children in low income families, who are nutritionally more vulnerable, are likely to watch more television, so this will be important in reducing inequalities.

- Commercial sponsorship of educational materials for schools needs to be controlled, so that commercial messages do not undermine healthy eating advice.

- Food skills should be compulsory in the national school curriculum, and initiatives for adults also need to be supported. The food skills of both adults and children – including budgeting, shopping, planning and cooking skills – need to be improved, to enable them to buy and prepare a healthy diet, and reduce dependence on pre-prepared and processed foods.

- Simple, easy-to-understand nutrition labelling should be introduced and there should be rigorous control of nutrition and health claims.

10 Local food strategies should be drawn up by local authorities, health authorities, industry and the voluntary sector, to address access and availability for low income groups. Targets should be set for all actors in the food chain.

Changes in food retailing patterns have led to a reduction in access to healthy food for poorer groups. Food retailing has become concentrated among large retailers, with two-thirds of produce now sold through supermarkets. Supermarkets now provide a wider variety of affordable healthy food than small local retailers. When available, food at local shops is, on average, 23% more expensive. However, an increasing number of supermarkets are out of town and therefore less accessible to low income families. A third of people in the UK do not have access to a car, and those in low income groups are least likely to have access to a car. Thus, healthy food is less available, and costs more, in deprived areas.

The issue of availability and access needs to be addressed by parallel strategies of making healthy food more available in poor areas, and improving access to larger shops.

A range of local initiatives are needed, with sustained funding. Health Improvement Programmes provide the framework for such local strategies; funding for Healthy Living Centres and Health Action Zones might be used for local food projects. Such a strategy could include the following:

- Addressing the issue of out-of-town shopping developments by refusing planning permission, or by making permission conditional on, for example, the provision of equivalent shelf space in poorer areas, or free bus services from low income areas to the shop.

- Incentives to support local shops selling good quality healthy food, and to encourage street markets and particularly vegetable and fruit stalls – especially in deprived areas. These could be encouraged by tax and rate rebates, differential rating or leasing tariffs, and security arrangements.

- An increase in the provision of free or subsidised allotments.

- Support and finance for local food initiatives, such as the formation of food co-operatives; new marketing strategies; and electronic networks to connect local shops to a central supply depot and improve access to a wider range of affordable foods.

Physical activity

11 The Department of Health, with other partners, should draw up and implement a national physical activity strategy which aims to integrate activity into daily life. The strategy should focus on children and should address transport, education and environment policies.

Physical inactivity is as important a risk factor for coronary heart disease as, for example, smoking or hypertension. The benefits of physical activity are graded: more activity, in terms of time and intensity, confers a greater health benefit. However, physical inactivity is more prevalent among the UK population than other risk factors. Exercise also plays an important part in coronary rehabilitation.

Patterns of physical activity vary between social groups: inequalities in levels of activity are clearly evident in relation to education, employment and housing tenure indicators, although social class indicators show mixed results.

These patterns are set early in life. Children from lower socioeconomic groups do less exercise on average than other children, particularly in out-of-school activity, although there are no social class differences in participation in school sports. Physical activity is more likely to be continued in adulthood if it is established as a regular activity in childhood.

The government has an important role in ensuring that transport, education and environment policies encourage physical activity as part of daily life, particularly for those from disadvantaged groups. The government should also set a minimum time for physical activity in the school curriculum as part of its focus on healthy schools.

12 Local authorities and health authorities should jointly develop local physical activity strategies, which include transport planning as well as leisure facilities.

Local authorities have an important role in ensuring provision for young people to continue to be physically active after they have left school, and as they make key transitions such as leaving further education, entering the labour market, and becoming parents. Such a strategy could include:

- concentrating high quality local authority sports and exercise provision in areas of socioeconomic deprivation, to increase opportunities for children and adults in lower income groups

- providing cheap and easy access to facilities, including subsidies and lower user charges, and provision of more facilities which are low-cost or free to users, such as football pitches and cycle lanes

- allocating a greater proportion of the transport budget to facilities which will encourage cycling and walking as part of people's daily routine. This will include addressing the quality of the physical environment, as well as safety issues.

13 Schools should introduce children to a wide range of activities and sports, in forms they enjoy.

Increased opportunities in school to participate in competitive and non-competitive sports encourage continuing participation in adulthood. Research also shows that the number of different activities to which a person is introduced is the best predictor of whether they continue in adulthood. Schools should provide opportunities, within and outside curriculum time, for children to participate in activity.

Psychosocial factors in the workplace

14 The government should produce a policy document on healthy work which recognises the health hazards of the psychosocial work environment, as well as the impact of the work environment on health behaviour, and the hazards of toxicological agents. This should inform the legal framework in the UK and the European Union, as well as company health and safety policies.

Improving the work environment is an important element of any strategy to reduce social inequalities in coronary heart disease. Importantly, what is good for health is also good for productivity, and therefore good for business. Effective interventions are available, but need to be implemented.

The threat to cardiovascular health at work is not only through exposure to traditional hazards such as smoking, but also to the psychosocial and organisational hazards of work – created by the design and management of organisations and work systems. Research shows a consistent positive association between poor psychosocial working conditions and increased coronary risk.

The three most important factors are: workload and the demands of work; the lack of control over individual working conditions, including the individual's ability to influence decisions; and the extent of social support in the workplace. Of these, control over work seems to be most important, explaining between 30% and 40% of the variance in coronary heart disease morbidity and mortality. Job strain – the combination of lack of control over work, and high psychological demands – in particular is associated with increased risk of coronary heart disease, and first heart attack. Other important factors in the workplace include the amount of reward given for job effort and the influence of shift work. Job insecurity has also been found to increase cardiovascular risk.

Health and safety legislation, in both the UK and the European Union (EU), places the duty on employers to ensure that work is 'safe and without risk to health'. Traditionally, these risks have been defined as physical but, with the new evidence, the definition needs to be broader. 'Healthy work' might be defined as 'work that maintains and enhances the physical, psychological and social health of the worker'. This definition should inform the legal framework as well as company policies and be used as a basis for all workplace health promotion programmes.

At a national level, there is a need for government policy or a policy statement on 'healthy work', perhaps within the context of existing health and safety regulations. This would help to legitimise the status of cardiovascular health as a workplace health and safety issue, and to demonstrate commitment to tackling the problem.

Legislation in the UK and the EU, which currently sets out minimum standards and general principles, and procedures for hazard reduction, could be extended to prescribe a comprehensive and detailed system of workplace controls for cardiovascular health.

National guidance on 'healthy work' policies is also needed to encourage organisations to develop their own policies. This might include guidance on: risk assessment and setting standards; workplace health promotion interventions; and education and training both within the workplace and of government advisers and inspectors. An outline policy document might be produced by the Health and Safety Commission, or Department of Health, for example.

15 **Employers should draw up and implement a policy on 'healthy work', including the organisation of work as well as more traditional health policies. This could be done within the context of the organisation's health and safety policy.**

While employers have a legal responsibility to assess work-related risks to the health and safety of employees, and to take reasonable action to reduce hazards, including the design and management of work, they currently have no statutory duty to support workplace health promotion activities, unless these are the appropriate response to an important health risk. Furthermore, risk assessment and reduction strategies have not yet been developed for psychosocial and organisational hazards.

Improvements to the psychosocial work environment need to include two interrelated approaches: addressing individual susceptibility to stress in terms of skills and abilities (perhaps through individual stress management programmes for employees), and the organisation of work and how it generates stress. A combined approach is likely to be most effective. Possibilities for improving the organisation of work include: increasing employees' authority over decisions which affect their working conditions; job rotation schemes; regular staff meetings; and the introduction of shifts which accommodate natural biological rhythms. Rewards are also important, and could be financial, or enhance a person's ability to control their work situation. Furthermore, as smokers experiencing 'job strain' find it harder to give up, initiatives which tackle both the job strain and the smoking will be important. Addressing job insecurity at an organisational and national level will also be important.

Workplace policies on healthy work might include, for example, a commitment to healthy work, standards and targets, guidance on hazard reduction and health promotion techniques, and organisational arrangements, as well as arrangements for monitoring and evaluation.

The 'in work' population is relatively easy to reach. However, the unemployed – and especially the 'never worked' population, and those whose participation in the workforce is marginal – now make up a substantial proportion of the population, and are particularly important in terms of health inequalities. It is inevitably harder to reach these groups and new strategies will be needed, perhaps under the auspices of the Social Exclusion Unit.

The role of the health service

16 **Health service strategies to reduce social class differences in coronary heart disease should be included in Health Improvement Programmes and Health Action Zones, and should form part of the National Service Framework for coronary heart disease.**

Health care provision does not seem to be a major cause of social inequalities in coronary heart disease, and is thus not the key to reducing health inequalities. While there are social class differentials in access to health services, it is difficult to demonstrate differentials in access that could account for the social class gradient in coronary heart disease mortality.

Firstly, there is little social class difference in the proportion of coronary patients who die at home, on the way to hospital, and in hospital, and any differences that do exist are too small to account for the social gradient in mortality. Secondly, research indicates that there is no social class difference in case fatality rates for coronary heart disease – that is, the proportion of hospital admissions which end in death. Thus, once a person is admitted to hospital with coronary heart disease, their chance of survival is not dependent on their social class.

However, improving health care could have an important impact on reducing rates of coronary disease among deprived social groups, to the extent that they are more likely to suffer from the disease. There is a clear relationship between deprivation and hospital admissions for coronary heart disease: those in deprived groups are 30% to 40% more likely to be admitted to hospital with coronary heart disease. Since about half of all coronary deaths occur in hospital, reducing hospital death rates will be particularly important, and could have an immediate impact on coronary death rates.

Options for action include:

- commitment of additional health service resources to local prevention strategies, particularly those of demonstrated effectiveness and those which tackle smoking

- inclusion of local smoking rates in the annual health service review process

- audit to assess and improve standards of hospital care and treatment, including thrombolytic therapy

- health centres employing or liaising with welfare benefit staff, to help improve knowledge and uptake of social benefits by low income families

- evaluation of the distribution and use of health promotion and disease prevention programmes in relation to need, to enable more effective planning and delivery, taking into account deprivation indices, levels of unemployment, psychosocial factors at work, and lifestyle factors, and

- greater liaison between GPs, nurses and voluntary groups, perhaps through Primary Care Groups, to develop a more proactive and community-oriented approach to health promotion, including monitoring.

Health Improvement Programmes, Health Action Zones, Primary Care Groups and Healthy Living Centres provide important vehicles to improve health service provision to reduce inequalities in coronary heart disease.

Research

17 Research funding bodies, including government, should ensure sustained funding for research on effective interventions to reduce inequalities in coronary heart disease, and highlight coronary heart disease as a focus for evaluated interventions to tackle health inequalities.

Research on inequalities in health has primarily focussed on the existence of such inequalities rather than on interventions to reduce them. Overall, there is a paucity of well designed intervention studies that address or measure social inequalities in coronary heart disease. What research has been done has tended to be small-scale and short-term.

There is a need for long-term investment in research on interventions aimed at reducing social inequalities in coronary heart disease, and evaluation of the impact of known, effective interventions on the health of different socioeconomic groups. Well designed, long-term studies are needed, preferably randomised controlled trials, which can be generalised to other settings. As the leading single cause of death, coronary heart disease could be used as a test case for interventions to reduce health inequalities.

In particular:

- Funding agencies could provide a powerful lead by requiring that socioconomic differences are measured in all research on coronary heart disease and risk factors, including epidemiology and interventions to reduce coronary risk. They could also require that evaluation is built into any initiatives aimed at reducing health inequalities.

- Researchers and NHS quality assurance programmes should examine the effects of interventions on different socioeconomic groups and, in particular, test known and effective interventions among different social groups.

- The government should undertake health impact assessments of the impact of different social and economic policies on coronary heart disease, and publish the results.

- The European Commission should establish health inequalities as a funding priority for public health to encourage European collaboration on the evaluation of interventions to reduce inequalities.

- There is a need for more research on the influence of deprivation and social inequalities across the life course, including income inequality, in order to establish their impact on health at different life stages, and the influences of exposure to deprivation in early and later life.

The Department of Health's research initiative on inequalities in health provides an important opportunity, with earmarked funds, to evaluate a range of interventions to reduce health inequalities, particularly those focussing on health determinants and on children and young people. It should be sustained over at least five years, and should highlight coronary heart disease as a focus for evaluated interventions to tackle health inequalities.

Reference

1   Department of Health. 1995. *Variations in Health: What Can the Department of Health and the NHS Do?* London: Department of Health.

While the recommendations set out in this chapter have considerable support, they do not necessarily reflect the specific views of all individual Forum member organisations or expert meeting participants.

Chapter 2

The magnitude of social inequalities in coronary heart disease: possible explanations

Professor Michael Marmot

International Centre for Health and Society, Department of Epidemiology and Public Health, University College London

Introduction

Coronary heart disease is a major health problem for the UK – a problem that cannot be dealt with adequately until social class differences in the disease have been addressed.

The issue of inequalities in coronary heart disease must be addressed, not only to increase understanding of the causes of the disease, but also in order to inform policy. There are two reasons for this. Firstly, it will be difficult to achieve the UK's targets for reducing coronary heart disease for the whole population if the health of only half of the population is improving. Secondly, there are ethical reasons for concern, since it is unacceptable to have such major differences in health status of different social groups of our population.

Despite recent improvements, the death rate from coronary heart disease in the UK is still among the highest in the world. It has recently been exceeded by some of the countries of Central and Eastern Europe where death rates have been rising rapidly. Although the death rate from coronary heart disease has been falling in the UK, it has not been falling as rapidly as in some other similar developed countries. If coronary heart disease were eliminated, life expectancy in the UK would increase by 4.7 years. Life expectancy would also be improved if all social groups in society were becoming healthier.[1]

The social gap in coronary heart disease mortality

There is a large social class gradient in coronary heart disease mortality rates, which is also reflected in premature death rates and morbidity from coronary heart disease, as well as in all cause mortality. Among men, the death rate from coronary heart disease is about 40% higher for those who are manual workers than for men who are non-manual workers. The rate for wives of manual workers is about twice as high as for the wives of non-manual workers.[2] This social class distribution of coronary heart disease has only been apparent in the last four decades. Until the early 1950s, in England and Wales, coronary heart disease was more common among social classes I and II. In the 1950s, however, a cross-over occurred, and since then, the disease has been more common in social classes IV and V.[3, 4]

There is also an increasing gap in health status between different social class groups for all cause mortality. Although mortality rates have fallen, it is the higher income groups that have the lower rates. Since 1972, there has been a decline in all cause mortality among men in all social class groups, except social class V. The social class difference in all cause standardised mortality ratios between social classes I and V has widened from an almost two-fold differential in 1970–1972 to an almost three-fold gap in 1991–1993 (see Figure 1).

The fact that the size of the gap changes over time and place shows that these variations are not fixed and that it might be possible to reduce them.

Figure 1 *All cause standardised mortality ratios by social class, at three time periods, men aged 20–64, England and Wales, 1970–1993*

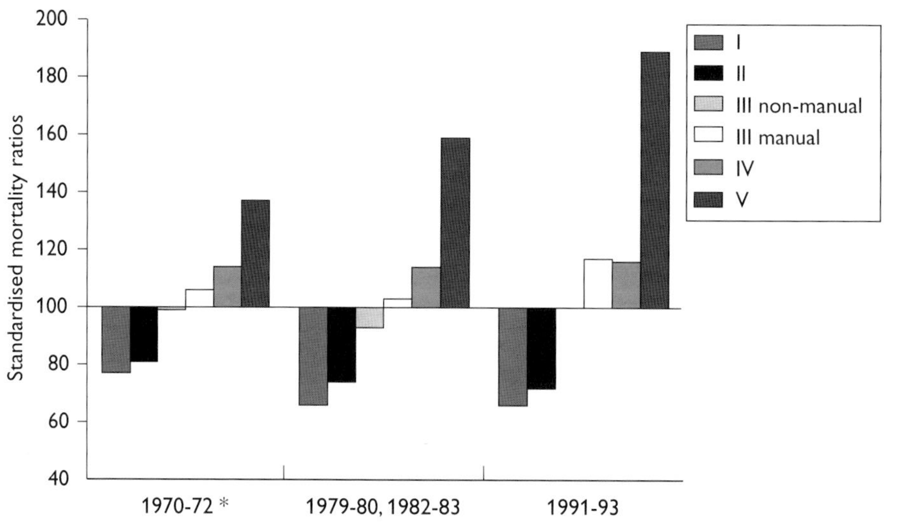

* Figures for 1970-72 are for age groups 15-64.

Source: See reference 5.

The social class gap in coronary heart disease mortality rates among men has also widened since the early 1970s, although for women the gap firstly narrowed and then widened again (see Figure 2). There has been a greater reduction in coronary heart disease death rates among non-manual groups than among manual groups. By the early 1990s, there was a three-fold difference in coronary heart disease mortality rates between professional (social class I) men and unskilled (social class V) men, from only a 25% excess in the early 1970s. This is the result of a small increase among social class V, but a huge reduction – a halving – in rates among social class I (see Figure 3). Thus the decline in mortality rates from coronary heart disease is largely due to reductions among non-manual groups.

The relationship between social deprivation and mortality varies across regions within the UK and may be independent of social class. That is to say, at equivalent levels of deprivation there are regional differences in mortality. This may, however, reflect differences in interpretation of the equivalent measurements of deprivation in different geographical regions.

Figure 2 *Age standardised death rates from coronary heart disease, men and women aged 35–64, by social class, 1976–1992*

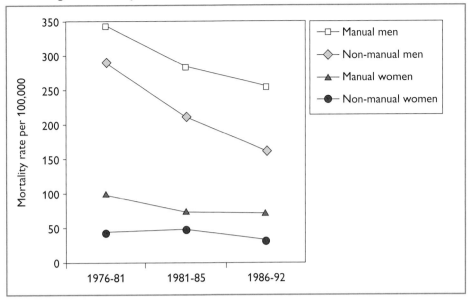

Source: See reference 6.

Figure 3 *Age standardised death rates from coronary heart disease, men aged 20–64, by social class, at three time periods, 1970–1993, England and Wales*

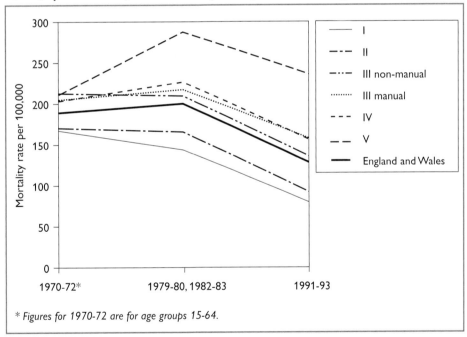

Source: See reference 5.

International comparisons

The problem of social inequalities in coronary heart disease rates is not unique to the UK. For example, mortality rates in the United States have been diverging between groups with high education and those with low education, among both white men and white women.[7]

There are also significant differences in:

- the magnitude of social class variations in coronary heart disease mortality rates within different countries, and

- coronary heart disease mortality and life expectancy between different countries.

These differences could provide some important clues about the nature of the mechanisms which might be operating.

The magnitude of social class variations within different countries

The magnitude of social class variations differs between European countries. For example, there is a markedly smaller variation in mortality rates between different social groups in Sweden, compared to the corresponding variation in the UK (see Figure 4). It must be recognised that the social class classifications are not identical. A recent investigation that attempted to deal with this issue confirmed that there are differences in the magnitude of social variations in diseases between countries.[8] This suggests that there are changeable causes that should be investigated.

Figure 4   All cause mortality rates by social class, men aged 20–64, England and Wales 1970–1972 and Sweden 1961–1979

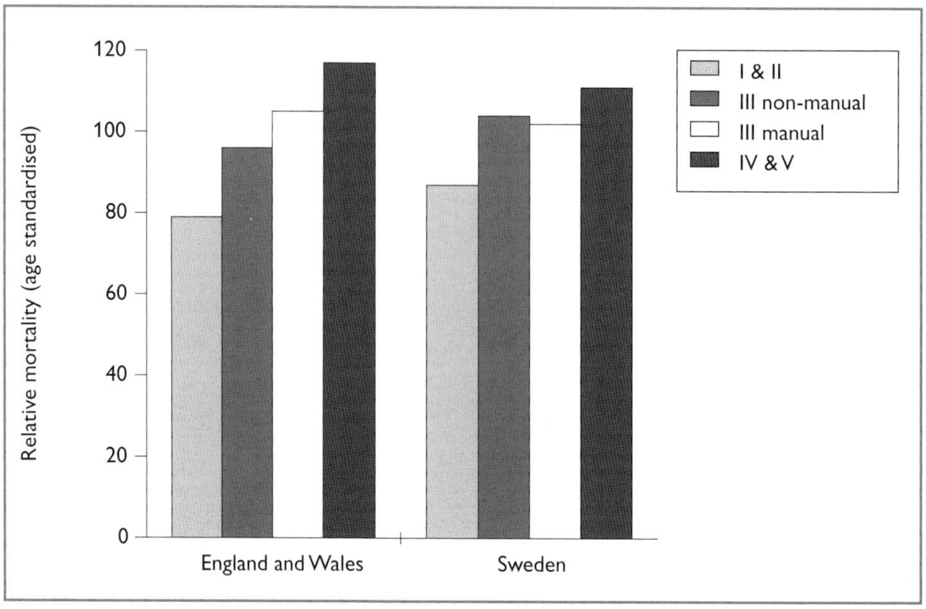

Source: See reference 9.

Coronary heart disease mortality and life expectancy in different countries

There are also significant differences in coronary heart disease mortality rates between different European countries. While these have been declining overall in Western Europe, in many Eastern European countries they have been rising[2] (see Figures 5 and 6).

Figure 5 Age standardised death rates from coronary heart disease, 1968–1994, selected Western European countries, men aged 35–74

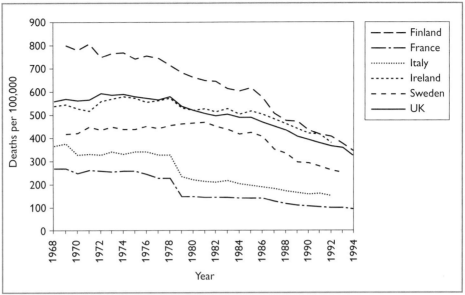

Source: See reference 2.

Figure 6 Age standardised death rates from coronary heart disease, 1968–1995, selected Central and Eastern European countries, men aged 35–74

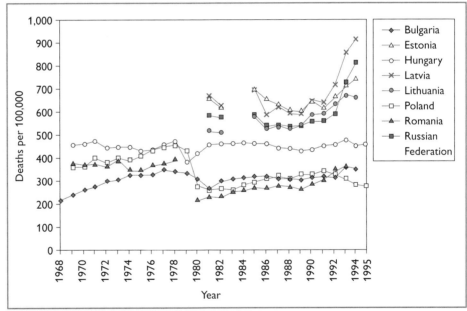

Source: See reference 2.

It is not simply that Central and Eastern Europeans are now dying of coronary heart disease instead of tuberculosis. Their life expectancy is not improving at the same rate as other European countries and, in some cases, is declining. Greater economic uncertainty and relative deprivation may be possible explanations. The poor economies of these countries since the 1970s contrast with the relative stability and wealth of the Western European nations. The psychosocial consequences of loss of cohesion as a result of relative deprivation may in part explain the higher rates of mortality. However, there is no simple explanation for the mortality gap between Eastern and Western Europe, and research to inform policy on the causes of such differences is needed.[10]

Income distribution

The pattern of income distribution within a country may have an important effect on health and life expectancy and may explain some of the variations in coronary heart disease mortality rates between countries. Countries with a relatively equitable income distribution tend to have longer life expectancy.[11]

Japan, which has the longest life expectancy in the world, also has the most egalitarian income distribution of all wealthy countries. In 1979, the poorest 20% of households in Japan had the highest proportion of total household income in any of the countries reported by the World Bank.[12]

The UK, with its lower life expectancy, has a less egalitarian income distribution. Although the wealth of Britons has increased over the last 20 years, the gap between high incomes and low incomes widened rapidly in the UK in the 1980s with an increasing proportion earning less than average income levels (see Figure 7). From 1977 to 1991, there was an almost continuous measurable rise in income inequality, although this has recently begun to level off.[13]

Figure 7 *Proportion of UK population below 40%, 50% and 60% of mean income, before housing costs, 1961–1991*

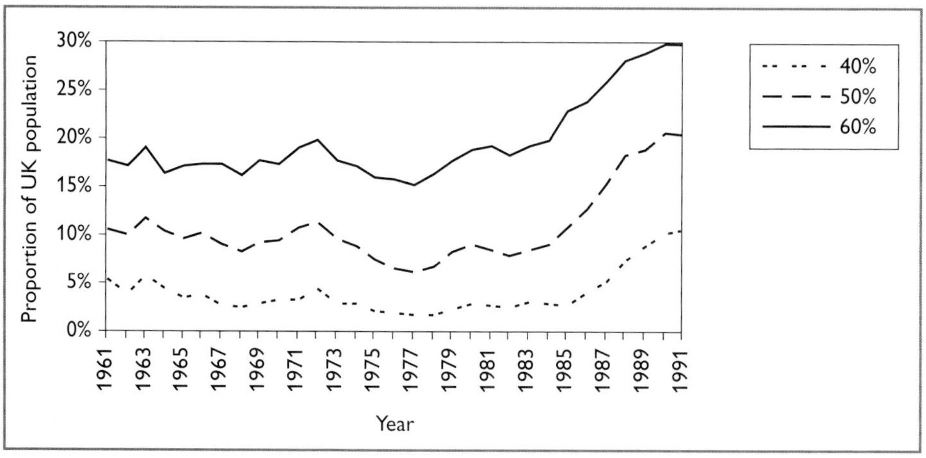

Source: See reference 13.

Not only did the rich become richer, but the poorest became poorer. Between 1979 and 1991/92 in the UK, the share of total income of the richest 20% (after housing costs) increased from 35.2% to 43%, while the share of the poorest 20% fell from 9.6% to 6.1%[14] (see Figure 8).

This trend is paralleled in the United States. Between 1977 and 1988, 80% of the population became poorer while the richest 20% increased their income by 16.5%. The top 5% had an increase of 23.4% and the top 1% approximately doubled their income.[15] The so-called trickle-down effects of economic policies favoured by the United States and the UK at the time benefited only a few.

Income differentials may be related to population health in two ways. Firstly, income differentials may be an indicator of the overall social environment that affects the health of the whole population; the greater the income differential, the greater the effect of the social environment on health. Secondly, the poorer the poor become, the worse their social conditions become and the poorer their health. Evidence suggests that income differentials are not necessary for economic growth.[16] There need, therefore, be no trade-off between economic policies and population health.

Figure 8 *Distribution of income by percentile of income, Great Britain, 1979 and 1991/1992 (after housing costs)*

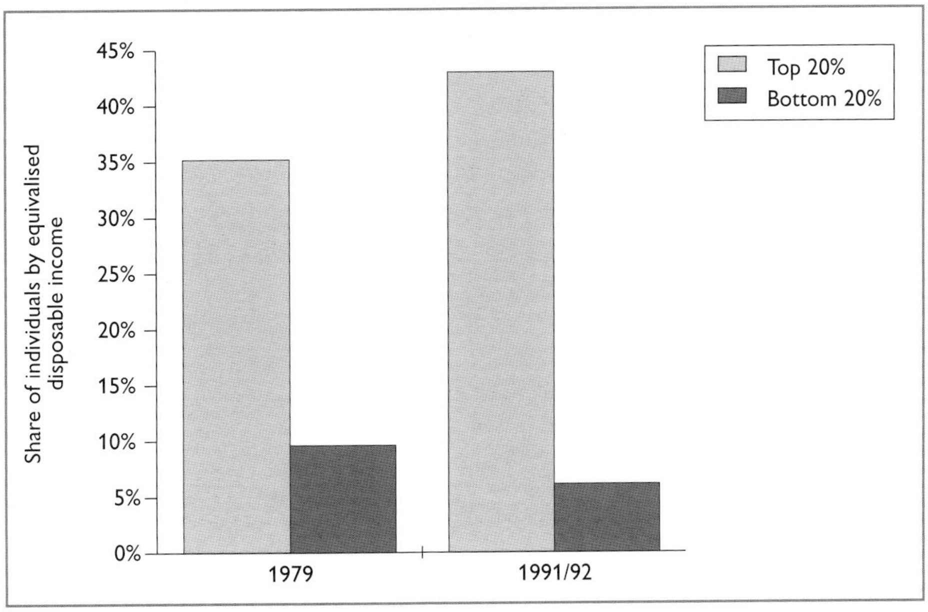

Source: See reference 14.

The gradient of social class inequalities

The social class variations in coronary heart disease reflect not just the contrast in material circumstances between the rich and the poor, but also the different psychosocial circumstances reflecting social position and the concomitant behavioural risks (such as smoking, diet and alcohol consumption).

The Whitehall I and II studies followed civil servants of different grades – administrators (the highest grade), professional and executive grades, and clerical grades and office support staff – for their subsequent experience of coronary heart disease. The Whitehall I study followed men over a 25-year period. Each grade in the civil service had a higher coronary heart disease mortality rate than the grade above it. Even though the lower grades are relatively poorly off, they are not poor in the absolute sense. There appears to be more ECG abnormality (an indicator of heart disease) among civil servants in the Whitehall I study compared to the Whitehall II study, but the social gradient in prevalence is undiminished.[17]

The social class gradient, clearly evident in the Whitehall studies, is not confined to the civil service. Similar gradients for all causes and for coronary heart disease are apparent across society.

The issue to be addressed is not only whether absolute poverty is related to ill health, but also how the relative differences in social position relate to the different risks of coronary heart disease and other diseases.

Possible explanations for social class inequalities in coronary heart disease

Several explanations for the social class differences in coronary heart disease have been proposed.

1 The health selection argument

One possible explanation is that it is not social position that determines health, but that health determines social position. People with poor health drift down the social hierarchy, or fail to move up. Evidence from the 1946[18] and 1958[19] birth cohorts and the OPCS longitudinal study[20] each showed that, while health has some effect on achieved social position, it is relatively minor and cannot account for the major social differentials in health in adulthood.

2 Behavioural factors

Research on coronary heart disease has concentrated on lifestyle and behavioural factors such as smoking, diet and physical activity. (See also Chapters 7–9.) Epidemiological research has been very successful in identifying risk factors that predict coronary heart disease; it is also important to examine how they relate to social inequalities.

Smoking

There is a striking social gradient in smoking. Among civil servants taking part in the Whitehall I survey, 29% of the top grades and 61% of the lowest grades smoked.[21] In the 20 years between the Whitehall I and Whitehall II studies, there was a significant decline in smoking. Although by 1985–88 (Whitehall II) the prevalence of smoking had decreased – to 9% of the top grades and 34% of the lower grades – the same social class gradient was reproduced.[17]

Smoking is a major preventable cause of premature morbidity and mortality. The persistent social class gradient in smoking is a cause for concern. It may be that the smoking problem in society as a whole cannot be solved without addressing the issue of social class gradient. This persisting social gradient may be exacerbated by health education programmes. If health education selectively reaches and influences some members of society more than others, it may increase the social differential in smoking. New policies may be needed.

Diet

The Whitehall II study revealed striking differences in consumption of fruit and vegetables between civil servants of different grades. Lower grade civil servants eat less fruit and vegetables.[17]

Social class differences in diet may be partly related to attitude and to having a sense of control over life. The percentage of civil servants who reported that they thought they could definitely reduce their risk of coronary heart disease was highest among the top grades. Those who thought they could definitely reduce their risk of heart attack were more likely to be eating a healthy diet (assessed by consumption of wholemeal bread, skimmed and semi-skimmed milk and fresh fruit and vegetables). They were three times more likely to eat a healthy diet than those who said they had no chance of reducing the risk of a heart attack. Thus, while behaviour is clearly important, health behaviour itself may be related to a belief in the ability to influence one's life, which in turn is related to social position.

The Dietary and Nutritional Survey of British Adults also found a marked social gradient in intake of fruit and vegetables.[22]

Physical activity
Although the effects of physical activity cannot yet be quantified from the Whitehall II study, there are social variations in patterns of physical activity. The lower grades take less exercise and are more likely to give up exercise as they get older. Among the high grades there is no decline with age in physical activity among the 35–55 year olds. Physical activity could be playing a role in the variations in coronary heart disease.[17]

Can behavioural factors explain the social variation in coronary heart disease?
Behavioural factors can explain only a small proportion of the variations in coronary heart disease risk between social groups.

In the Whitehall I study, there was a 2.7-fold variation in the relative risk of coronary heart disease death, over a 10-year period, between the highest and lowest employment grades in the civil service. When differences in age, smoking, blood pressure, cholesterol level, height, and blood sugar are adjusted for, the variation in relative risk reduces to 2.2 (see Figure 9).

Figure 9   *Relative risk of coronary heart disease death in 10 years, controlling for age and other risk factors*

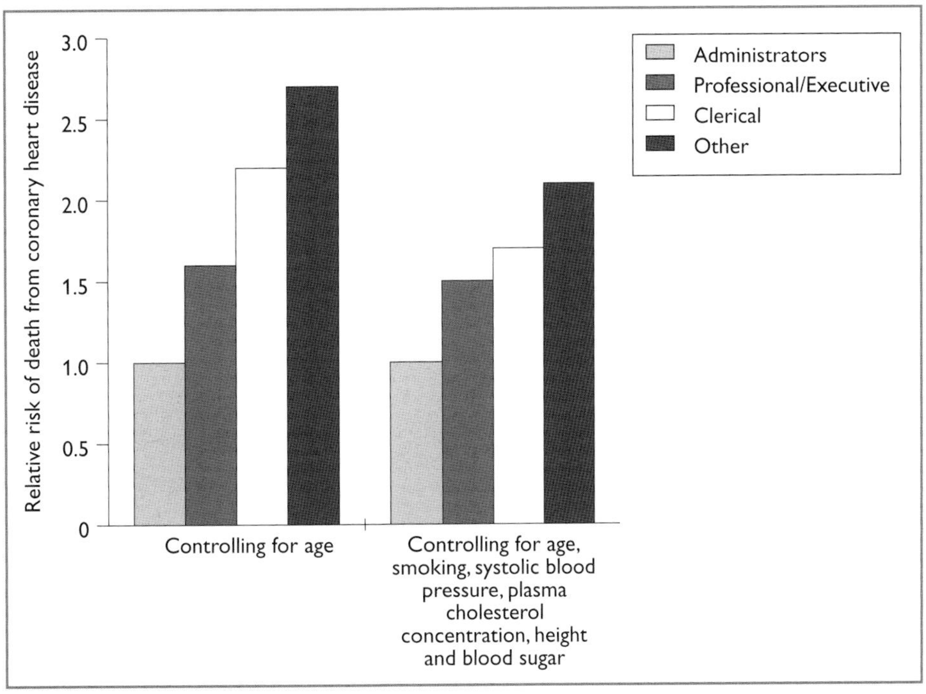

Source: See reference 21.

Although Whitehall I found a lower risk of coronary heart disease in the higher grades, plasma cholesterol levels were marginally higher in higher grades and there were only small differences in blood pressure between grades. The gradient of coronary heart disease mortality risk was also identical among smokers and non-smokers. The well-known risk factors for coronary heart disease thus do not appear to explain the bulk of the social class differences.[21]

Behavioural risk factors cannot explain the variation in coronary heart disease between countries either. Differentials in mortality between Eastern European countries and Western European countries cannot be explained by smoking or plasma cholesterol levels.[23] While cholesterol is a major determinant of coronary risk in individuals, differences in mean plasma cholesterol bear very little relationship to the variation in coronary heart disease mortality between Central and Eastern Europe and Western Europe.[10] A large proportion of the variation in coronary heart disease both within and between countries thus remains unexplained by health behaviour.

3 Material differences

While civil service grades relate to status, they also relate closely to income. Different social class groups have different material circumstances which may explain the differences in risk of coronary heart disease. It is not yet known if material conditions, such as living in a two-bedroomed flat or a five-bedroomed house, affect an individual's risk of coronary heart disease.

4 Early life factors

There is increasing evidence to suggest that what happens in the womb and in the first year of life may be an important determinant of coronary heart disease risk in middle age. There appears to be a relationship between smaller size at birth and weight at one year, and increased risk of coronary heart disease. Smaller size at birth is linked to four coronary heart disease risk factors: raised blood pressure, non-insulin dependent diabetes, raised serum cholesterol and high plasma fibrinogen concentrations.[24] Although early influences may be important, it is most likely that what happens after the age of one year still has a very important influence on coronary heart disease risk in adulthood.

The height differentials between civil servants were examined in the Whitehall II study as one indicator of conditions in early life. Height is determined by genes and environment, and presumably early life environment. There is a clear relationship between height and employment grade: men and women in the higher grades tend to be taller.

Findings from the Whitehall I study showed that height predicted mortality independently of current grade of employment, that is to say shorter people had a higher risk of coronary heart disease, regardless of their grade.[21] However, employment grade also predicts mortality independently of height.

Thus there are two independent predictors: height and current social position. In other words, a healthy early life environment does not give protection from the adverse effects of social status on health.

5 Plasma fibrinogen levels

Haemostatic factors, another potential explanatory factor for the social class gradient in coronary heart disease, show an inverse gradient by grade of employment in both men and women in the Whitehall II study. Recent research has found an inverse relation between plasma fibrinogen concentration and socioeconomic status in middle-aged men and women; the lower the grade, the higher the plasma fibrinogen.[25] Factors operating throughout life may influence adult fibrinogen concentration and thereby the risk of coronary heart disease.[26]

6 Psychosocial factors

It is plausible that relative material differences might operate through psychosocial mechanisms such as low self-esteem or chronic stress. However, they explain only a small proportion of the variation.

One way to examine the effect of psychosocial factors on coronary heart disease risk is to look at sickness absence rates among civil servants, as these rates differ considerably between grades. Smoking, aspects of the psychosocial work environment, psychiatric symptoms, aspects of the social environment outside work (such as social support), financial problems and ethnic group all predict sickness absence. However, even after adjustment for these factors, there still remains a gradient of sickness absence across the grades.[27]

The psychosocial work environment and the social environment outside work are potentially important mediators of the link between social position and health, but much more research needs to be done.

7 Access to health care

It is difficult to demonstrate differentials in access to health care that could account for the social class gradient in coronary heart disease mortality. Although there is a two-fold difference in the 'consumption of health care' between social classes, this does not appear to explain the three-fold difference in mortality that is apparent between the lowest and highest employment grades of the civil service.

Conclusion

There is no longer any doubt that social class differences in coronary heart disease rates do exist. There is now a need to address why they exist, to uncover the factors which mediate between social status, income and ill health and, armed with this information, to address them in policy terms. For all those involved in public health, the question is 'What can we do about the social class differences in coronary heart disease?'

References

1   Marmot MG, Davey Smith G. 1989. Why are the Japanese living longer? *British Medical Journal*; 299: 1547–1551.

2   Kaduskar S, Bradshaw H, Rayner M. 1997. *Coronary Heart Disease Statistics*. London: British Heart Foundation.

3   Marmot MG, McDowall ME. 1986. Mortality decline and widening social inequalities. *Lancet*; ii: 274–276.

4   Marmot MG, Adelstein AM, Robinson N, Rose GA. 1987. Changing social class distribution of heart disease. *British Medical Journal*; 2: 1109–1112.

5   Drever F, Whitehead M, Roden M. 1996. Current patterns and trends in male mortality by social class based on occupation. *Population Trends*; 86: 15–20.

6   Drever F, Whitehead M. 1997. *Health Inequalities: Decennial Supplement*. London: The Stationery Office.

7   Pattas G, Queen S, Hadden W, Fisher G. 1993. The increasing disparity in mortality between socioeconomic groups in the United States, 1960 and 1986. *New England Journal of Medicine*; 329: 103–109.

8   Mackenbach JP, Kunst AE, Covelaars AE, Grorenhof F, Geurts JJ. 1997. Socioeconomic inequalities in morbidity and mortality in Western Europe. The EU Working Group on Socioeconomic Inequalities in Health. *Lancet*; 349: 1655-1659.

9   Vagero D, Lundgren O. 1989. Health inequalities in Britain and Sweden. *Lancet*; 299: 35–36.

10   Bobak M, Marmot MG. 1996. East-West mortality divide and its potential explanations: proposed research agenda. *British Medical Journal*; 312: 421–425.

11   Wilkinson R. 1996. *Unhealthy Societies: The Afflictions of Inequality*. London: Routledge.

12   Office of Health Economics. 1987. *Compendium of Health Statistics. 6th edition*. London: Office of Health Economics.

13   Goodman A, Webb S. 1994. *For Richer, for Poorer: The Changing Distribution of Income in the United Kingdom, 1961–1991*. London: Institute of Fiscal Studies.

14   Joseph Rowntree Foundation. 1995. *Joseph Rowntree Foundation Inquiry into Income and Wealth. Volume 2*. York: Joseph Rowntree Foundation.

15   Phillips K. 1990. *The Politics of Rich and Poor*. New York: Random House.

16   World Bank. 1993. *The East Asian Miracle*. Oxford: Oxford University Press.

17   Marmot MG, Davey Smith G, Stansfeld S, Patel C, North F, Head J, White I, Brunner E, Feeney A. 1991. Health inequalities among British civil servants: the Whitehall II study. *Lancet*; 337: 1387–1393.

18   Wadsworth MEJ. Serious illness in childhood and its association with later life achievement. In: Wilkinson R (ed.) *Class and Health*: 50-74. London: Tavistock Publications.

19   Power C, Manor O, Fox J. 1991. *Health and Class: The Early Years*. London: Chapman and Hall.

20   Fox J, Goldblatt P, Jones D. Social class mortality differentials: selection or life circumstances? In: Goldblatt P (ed.) 1990. *Longitudinal Mortality and Social Organisation*. London: HMSO.

21   Marmot MG, Rose G, Shipley MJ. 1984. Inequalities in death – specific explanations of a general pattern. *Lancet*; 305: 1003–1006.

22   Ministry of Agriculture, Fisheries and Food. 1994. *The Dietary and Nutritional Survey of British Adults – Further Analysis*. London: HMSO.

23   Bobak M, Hense HW, Kark J, Kuch B, Vojtisek P, Sinnreich R, Gostomzyk J, Bui M, von Eckardstein A, Junker R, Fobker M, Schulte H, Assman G, Marmot M. 1997. Explaining cardiovascular disease rate differences: risk factors in Czech, Bavarian and Israeli men. Submitted.

24   Barker DJP. 1995. Fetal origins of coronary heart disease. *British Medical Journal*; 311: 171–174.

25   Brunner EJ, Marmot MG, White IR, O'Brien JR, Etherington MD, Slavin BM, Kearney EM, Davey Smith G. 1993. Gender and employment grade differences in blood cholesterol, apolipoproteins and haemostatic factors in the Whitehall II study. *Atherosclerosis*; 102: 195–207.

26   Brunner E, Davey Smith G, Marmot M, Canner R, Beksinska M, O'Brien J. 1996. Childhood social circumstances and psychosocial and behavioural factors as determinants of plasma fibrinogen. *Lancet*; 347: 1008–13.

27   North F, Syme SL, Feeney A, Head J, Shipley MJ, Marmot MG. 1993. Explaining socioeconomic differences in sickness absence: the Whitehall II study. *British Medical Journal*; 306: 361–366.

Professor Michael Marmot is an individual member of the National Heart Forum.

Chapter 3

Influences through the life course: from early life to adulthood

Professor George Davey Smith

Department of Social Medicine, University of Bristol

Introduction

There are large social class inequalities in mortality from all the major cardiovascular diseases including coronary heart disease and stroke, and also in all cause mortality, among men and women of working ages in the UK.[1] (These inequalities are described in greater detail in Chapter 2.) This socioeconomic distribution is also seen in morbidity rates. For example, in a survey of over 20,000 people aged 35 and over in Somerset and Avon, histories of angina, myocardial infarction (heart attack), and stroke were all more common among individuals living in deprived compared to affluent areas[2] (see Table 1). Socioeconomic position is also related to the early stages of developing cardiovascular disease. For example, in a Finnish study, low income, manual occupation and little education were all related to a higher severity of carotid atherosclerosis.[3]

Until recently the debate regarding inequalities in health generally related to the association of illness with socioeconomic circumstances in adulthood. There has recently been a revival of interest in the effects of poor social circumstances in early life on health in adulthood.[4, 5] The UK Department of Health report, *Variations in Health*,[6] has recognised the importance of a life course perspective on inequalities in health. It concludes that it "is likely that accumulative differential lifetime exposure to health-damaging or health-promoting physical and social environments is the main explanation for observed variations in health and life expectancy".

Table I *Age standardised prevalence per 100 of self-reported illness by deprivation category*

Condition	1st fifth (least deprived)	2nd fifth	3rd fifth	4th fifth	5th fifth (most deprived)	P value (test for trend)
Men						
Angina	4.4	5.5	5.5	5.5	6.9	<0.001
Myocardial infarction	3.2	3.7	4.0	4.5	4.8	<0.001
Stroke	2.0	1.8	1.3	2.3	2.6	0.03
Women						
Angina	3.8	4.4	4.6	4.4	5.8	<0.002
Myocardial infarction	1.5	1.9	1.7	1.8	2.5	0.03
Stroke	1.6	2.0	2.1	2.2	2.4	0.04

Source: See reference 2.

The cumulative effect of socioeconomic position at different stages of life

There are few empirical data regarding cumulative effects of socioeconomic position at different stages in the life course. In a cohort study which followed men for over 20 years in the west of Scotland,[7,8] it was possible to relate mortality experience to three factors:
– the social class of the fathers of the men
– the social class of the first occupation of the men on entering the labour market, and
– the social class of their occupation at the time of screening, when aged 35–64.

It has been demonstrated that cumulative social class – indexed simply by summing the manual and non-manual social class locations at the three stages of the life course – together with other indicators of socioeconomic position at the time of screening are strongly related to mortality risk[8] (see Table 2). When social class at different periods of the life course is related to mortality from specific causes, two factors independently contribute to all cause and cardiovascular mortality:
– social class of the fathers of the men, and
– their own social class at the time of screening.

This indicates that there are some long-lasting influences of socioeconomic circumstances in childhood on mortality in adulthood.

Table 2 *All cause mortality by cumulative social class, car ownership and deprivation category*

Age adjusted relative rates

	Cumulative social class*			
	All 3 non-manual	2 non-manual and 1 manual	2 manual and 1 non-manual	All 3 manual
Car	1	1.28 (1.01, 1.63)	1.36 (1.08, 1.73)	1.57 (1.27, 1.95)
No car	1.22 (0.91, 1.64)	1.52 (1.19, 1.95)	1.76 (1.40, 2.21)	2.00 (1.64, 2.44)
Deprivation category 1–4	1	1.25 (1.01, 1.56)	1.37 (1.09, 1.72)	1.70 (1.39, 2.09)
Deprivation category 5–7	1.06 (0.74, 1.52)	1.41 (1.10, 1.82)	1.54 (1.25, 1.90)	1.74 (1.45, 2.09)

* Cumulative social class is indexed by summing the manual and non-manual class locations at the three stages of the life course.

Source: See reference 8.

The suggestion that mortality risk reflects the accumulation of environmental 'insults' (adverse events or circumstances) across the life course, or the cumulative effects of unfavourable behavioural or psychological factors which progressively increase susceptibility to disease,[9, 10] receives further support from a study based on the 1960, 1970 and 1980 census records for Norway. In this study, particularly high mortality risks are seen among men who had limited education and then went on to work in manual occupations and live in poor housing.[11] Similar findings have come from the National Longitudinal Study of older men in the United States.[12] Childhood socioeconomic circumstances make a particular contribution to cardiovascular disease risk. This has been demonstrated in the Scottish cohort discussed above,[7] and also in area-based studies from Finland, which indicate that the association between childhood socioeconomic circumstances and cardiovascular risk is stronger than the association between childhood circumstances and other causes of death.[13, 14]

Socioeconomic circumstances in childhood and adulthood have been examined with respect to a variety of cardiovascular disease risk factors in the Scottish cohort mentioned above.[15] Cigarette smoking was more common among men in manual than in non-manual occupations, with father's social class contributing little to the distribution of smoking behaviour when examined in addition to the social class of the men themselves. This suggests that smoking behaviour is determined by current social environment, rather than by any particular influences of childhood environment. In contrast, height is associated both with father's social class and with own adulthood social class. This could reflect environmental – particularly nutritional – effects from early life, together with the possible contribution of height-related upward social mobility. Body mass index was more strongly associated with father's social class than own social class, with the reverse being the case for blood pressure and cholesterol levels. Fibrinogen was not measured in the Scottish cohort, but in the Whitehall II study fibrinogen levels were associated with indicators of both parental social class and of current socioeconomic position.[16]

Thus, experiences at different stages of the life course appear to make specific contributions to particular cardiovascular disease risk factors. One nutritional factor which may contribute to the life course accumulation of disease risk is that of fruit and vegetable intake.[17] In a study of Finnish men, intakes of fruit, non-root vegetables and vitamin C were related to childhood socioeconomic circumstances,[18] implying that this adult dietary behaviour may become established early in life and may not be readily amenable to change at a later stage.

Factors in early life

The question 'What are the long-term effects of development during foetal and early infant life on disease risk in adulthood?' is of particular current research interest. Although several early studies had highlighted the importance of early-life factors in later disease risk,[4, 5, 19, 20] interest in early influences on adult cardiovascular disease mortality was regenerated by the work of Forsdahl[21] who related infant mortality rates in Norway earlier this century to present day coronary heart disease mortality rates.

Forsdahl demonstrated that, in areas where infant mortality rates had been high in the past and where, by implication, children had been nutritionally deprived both in early infancy and in childhood, coronary heart disease mortality rates 70 years later were also high. While these data are suggestive, it is precisely those places which had high infant mortality rates at the beginning of this century which remain the most deprived places today. If current deprivation levels are taken into account in the analysis, there is essentially no residual association between past infant mortality rates and present coronary heart disease mortality rates[22] (see Figure 1). While these data do not mean that early life factors have no importance, they do demonstrate the need for studies with adequate data across the life course if the separate effects of early life and later life exposures are to be ascertained.

Since the pioneering work of Forsdahl, a series of studies have demonstrated that birth weight and weight at one year of age are inversely related to cardiovascular disease, diabetes and blood pressure in later life.[23] These findings support the proposition that there are important persisting influences of development in early life on cardiovascular disease risk in adulthood. Further studies, with adequate data across the life course, are needed to take this area of research forward.

In recent years little research has been carried out on the effects of childhood nutrition on later disease, although earlier this century it was considered obvious that such effects did exist.[4, 5] Preliminary data are now available from a mortality follow-up of the children included in surveys of poverty, nutrition and child health carried out under the auspices of Lord John Boyd Orr in the period immediately before the Second World War.[24]

At the time this survey was carried out, one of the investigators recognised that leg length was a particularly good indicator of childhood socioeconomic and nutritional circumstances:

"When the Carnegie UK Dietary and Clinical Survey was planned at the Rowett Research Institute in 1937, cristal height as a measurement of leg length was included in the measurements ... it was found that cristal height was consistently better than total height for indicating expenditure group ... we find the longer-legged children suffered less bronchitis than the short at all ages. Since there is neither complicating immunity mechanism nor specific cure for bronchitis, we might argue that constitution built up when the complete harmonious pattern of growth is unfolded is, in some way, superior to that associated with inhibition of growth, however slight."[25]

Figure 1   Infant mortality rates 1905–1908 and female coronary heart disease mortality age 65–74 in 1969–1973, before and after control for measure of adult deprivation

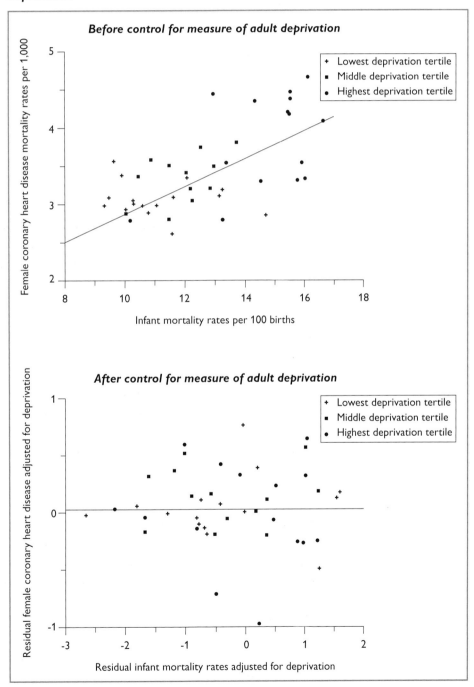

Source: See reference 22.

In a re-analysis of these data, this is clearly the case[26] (see Table 3). Age standardised indicators of total height, leg length and trunk length reveal differential associations with nutritional and socioeconomic factors. It is particularly noticeable that the negative correlations between overcrowding and social class of head of household (scored from 1 for professional groups to 5 for unskilled manual workers) are considerably stronger for leg length than for trunk length. The positive correlations between weighted per capita food expenditure and relative family per capita calorie consumption are also stronger for leg length than trunk length. The results for females and males are similar.

Table 3 *Relationship between anthropometric, childhood dietary and socioeconomic factors and adult socioeconomic status, in males*

Anthropometric, dietary or socioeconomic index *(n)*	Height *'z' score*	Leg length *'z' score*	Trunk length *'z' score*
Birth order *(1,397)*	−0.14	−0.14	−0.06
Number of children *(1,394)*	−0.25	−0.24	−0.14
Weighted per capita food expenditure *(1,394)*	0.31	0.33	0.14
Social class of head of household *(1,287)*	−0.18	−0.21	−0.05
Overcrowding *(1,220)*	−0.19	−0.20	−0.08
Relative family per capita calorie consumption *(1,394)*	0.23	0.26	0.08

This table uses Pearson's correlation coefficient.

Source: See reference 26.

Leg length in childhood is associated with mortality over the subsequent 60 years, as Table 4 shows. These data suggest that childhood nutrition may have important long-term consequences on health in later life. They do not, however, paint a one-sided view of rapid growth in childhood. In line with evidence from animal studies and some epidemiological findings,[27, 28] they suggest that cancer risk may be increased by greater calorie intake and growth in early life. Thus reductions in cardiovascular disease mortality in response to socioeconomic and nutritional conditions which encourage growth in childhood may, in part, be counter-balanced by increases in cancer mortality.

The ratio of leg length to total height changes throughout childhood, but those children with a high ratio are likely to become adults with a high ratio. Thus it is possible to investigate the association between leg length in adulthood and the risk of cardiovascular disease, using the former in part as a proxy for exposures during childhood. The Caerphilly study [29] related sitting height and leg length with 10-year follow-up data on coronary heart disease incidence and mortality. Coronary heart disease risk is inversely associated with leg length and with the ratio of leg length to sitting height, whereas the association with overall height is weak. Furthermore, the components of syndrome X – insulin resistance, high fasting triglyceride levels, low HDL cholesterol and obesity – are more common among the men with shorter legs and with low leg length to sitting height ratios. This suggests that development during childhood may be related to the risk of syndrome X, which in turn increases cardiovascular disease risk.[30]

Table 4   Leg length and mortality in the Carnegie survey follow-up

Quintile	Coronary heart disease mortality Fully adjusted relative risk (*95% confidence interval)	Cancer mortality Fully adjusted relative risk (*95% confidence interval)
Males		
1 (shortest)	2.8 (1.1, 6.9)	0.4 (0.1, 1.1)
2	2.5 (1.0, 6.0)	0.4 (0.2, 1.1)
3	2.2 (0.9, 5.2)	0.6 (0.2, 1.5)
4	2.5 (1.1, 5.7)	0.8 (0.4, 1.8)
5 (tallest)	1.0	1.0
Linear trend test	p = 0.09	p = 0.06
Females		
1 (shortest)	4.2 (0.8, 22.2)	1.0 (0.4, 2.3)
2	3.5 (0.7, 17.8)	1.1 (0.5, 2.4)
3	1.9 (0.3, 10.6)	1.0 (0.4, 2.2)
4	0.9 (0.1, 6.6)	0.8 (0.4, 2.0)
5 (tallest)	1.0	1.0
Linear trend test	p = 0.006	p = 0.77

* Adjusted for age and indices of childhood and adult socioeconomic circumstances, calorie consumption, and birth order

Source: See reference 26.

Writing in 1951, Isabella Leitch discussed what happened to animals which were stunted at birth due to poor nutrition, but were then well fed during later life. She discussed a particular animal model that she used in her work which she called the 'low-high pig', stunted in growth and becoming obese 'rather than finished' when it is then well fed.[25] She postulated that this is what would happen to children who were poorly nourished in childhood but given a more calorific diet in later life. Data showing that obesity is more strongly related to childhood than adulthood socioeconomic circumstances give support to this hypothesis.[15]

Studies of birthweight and cardiovascular disease risk factors have suggested that interactions may occur between early life and later life exposures. A Swedish study, for example, demonstrated that low birthweight babies who became obese adults had high blood pressure and high rates of insulin resistance.[31] In the Caerphilly study, birthweight is inversely related to risk of coronary heart disease in adulthood.[29] This association is robust when adjustment is made for a wide range of conventional cardiovascular disease risk factors. However, the relationship between birthweight and coronary heart disease risk is restricted to men in the highest body mass index tertile in adulthood.[32] Similarly, the association between leg length and leg to sitting height ratio and coronary heart disease risk is strongest among the men who became obese in adult life.

Recent research has demonstrated important interactions between socially patterned exposures in early life – such as low birthweight and poor growth – and later life exposures, reflected in obesity levels. Studies of how factors accumulating and interacting over the life course generate cardiovascular disease risk are still in their infancy, but offer to advance our understanding of how social phenomena are translated into socioeconomic inequalities in cardiovascular disease risk.

Education

There is also emerging evidence of the important role of education in the life cycle, as a determinant of health. Research in the United States points to health gains in adult life, which are linked to educational and social interventions in childhood. Programmes in the post-neonatal, pre-school and school-age periods, often involving both parents and children, are believed to have positive effects on cognitive and social-emotional development. These, in turn, could improve long-term outcomes in health, well-being and competence throughout the life cycle.[33]

In the UK, an observational study found that both education and social class can serve as indices of life course socioeconomic experience, and both are strongly associated with mortality in middle-aged men. Cardiovascular disease is the cause of death which was most strongly associated with a low level of education, which could reflect that education is an indicator of socioeconomic circumstances in childhood. Education is likely to be important for the opportunities it creates for improved material conditions of life, rather than for specific effects of education itself.[34]

There is also evidence that people with low educational qualifications and attainment are least likely to respond to health education messages, such as those relating to smoking and diet. This may be due to a variety of factors, such as the association of poor education with low income and consequent access to a healthy diet, or peer group influences.[35] Adult social class is more strongly associated with smoking than is education, indicating the importance of adulthood social environment in determining the distribution of smoking behaviour.[34] Improving levels of education is potentially an important way of improving population health. This is only the case, however, when better education provides access to more favourable social environments throughout life.

Factors in adulthood

Several studies have investigated the contribution of particular health-related behaviours and physiological risk factors to differentials in mortality.

In the first Whitehall study of London civil servants, considerable differences were found in mortality risk according to two socioeconomic measures – employment grade in the civil service and car ownership. Car ownership was a good indicator of available income in the late 1960s, when this study was established.[36] While smoking behaviour was patterned such that the lower grade and non-car owning civil servants were more likely to smoke than the higher grade and car owning ones, the pattern of differentials in all cause mortality among men who had never smoked was identical to that of the whole cohort.[37, 38]

There was a very similar association of cardiovascular disease mortality with employment grade and car ownership (see Figure 2), as there was for all cause mortality. However, cholesterol levels were greater among higher rather than lower grade civil servants in the late 1960s, when this study was established. Therefore, the differences in cholesterol levels could not account for the higher rates of coronary heart disease among the lower grade employees. This seems to suggest that differences in dietary fat intake between grades were not responsible for the coronary heart disease mortality differentials. Indeed, a whole range of risk factors – including smoking, blood pressure, cholesterol levels and prevalent cardiorespiratory disease – failed to account for the grade differences in cardiovascular and non-cardiovascular mortality between the different grades of employees.[36]

Figure 2 *Cardiovascular disease mortality by employment grade and car ownership in the Whitehall Study*

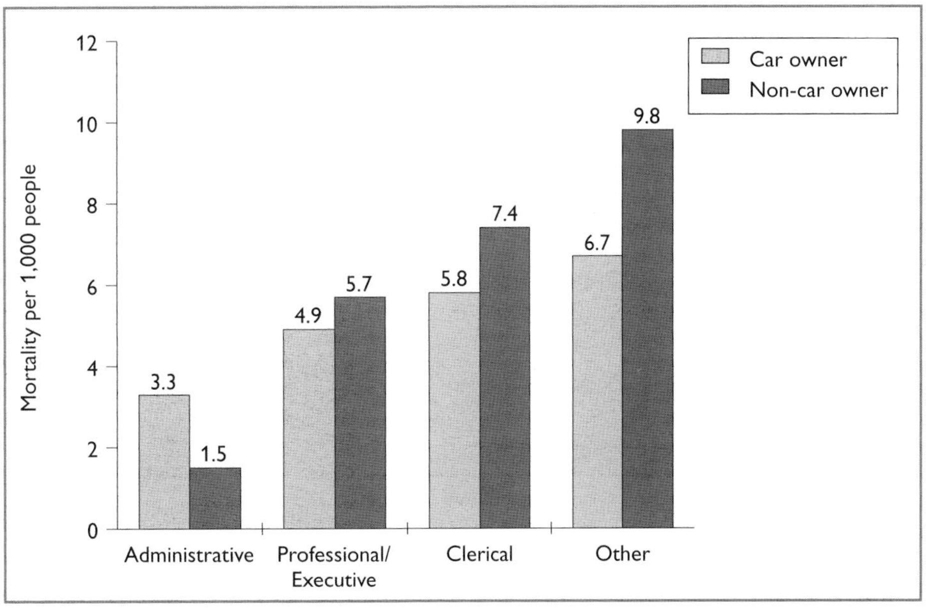

Source: See reference 36.

Similar findings have emerged from a study in the West of Scotland established at about the same time as the first Whitehall study.[7,8] In the Scottish study, there were large differentials in cardiovascular disease mortality according to both father's and own social class, at a time when blood cholesterol levels were highest in those with professional and managerial occupations. Adjustments for a wide range of risk factors failed to explain the considerable differentials in mortality from cardiovascular disease.

These findings are not limited to British studies. A prospective study of one-third of a million men screened for the Multiple Risk Factor Intervention Trial in the United States between 1970 and 1973, with 16 years of mortality follow-up, found a strong association between the income level of the area of residence of the men and their risk of mortality from coronary heart disease and stroke.[39,40] Although adjustments for smoking, cholesterol levels, blood pressure and diabetes reduced these associations to some extent, they did not remove them.

As conventional risk factors had failed to account adequately for the social distribution of cardiovascular disease, the Whitehall II study was initiated in 1985 to explore additional psychosocial, behavioural, dietary and metabolic factors which could contribute to the socioeconomic differentials in health. The baseline examinations showed a lower prevalence of cardiorespiratory disease among higher grade civil servants – with higher incomes – among both sexes.[41] Average cholesterol levels were similar in each grade, but concentrations of serum apolipoprotein AI, the main structural protein of HDL cholesterol, showed an association with grade.[42] This suggested that characteristic disturbances of lipid metabolism associated with lower occupational status could potentially be identified.

An opportunistic study using data from the Whitehall II civil servants cohort examined the effect of job insecurity on health status. When the baseline examinations were carried out in the mid-1980s, the civil servants thought they had secure jobs for life. Partly as a response to the initiatives implemented following the reviews of civil service efficiency introduced by Lord Rayner, privatisation of some civil service functions was discussed and later implemented. The first civil service department to experience these changes was the Property Services Agency (PSA). From 1988 on it became clear that changes were to be made to the PSA and that jobs were therefore insecure. By 1993 the PSA was fully privatised. The rest of the civil service remained a relatively secure employer, at least until 1990. Thus the health of the group of people undergoing the stress associated with the anticipation, and then the reality, of their employment being rationalised, could be examined in relation to the control group.

At the time of the repeat examinations in 1990, PSA workers, who had generally better health at the time of the baseline examinations than the rest of the cohort, were reporting more symptoms of ill health, and worse overall health over the previous year.[43] Two years later, clinical examinations were repeated when the PSA employees were actually experiencing rationalisation, privatisation and loss of secure employment. Cholesterol levels and body mass index in men and women had increased in the PSA compared to those in the other civil service departments. There was an increase in blood pressure for women and a non-significant increase in coronary heart disease for men and women combined.

These effects suggest a higher risk of cardiovascular disease among members of the first civil service agency to experience privatisation, and the study demonstrates how a particular form of social stress could increase cardiovascular disease risk. Further work of high methodological quality on the effects of psychosocial stress on risk of disease is required, since much research in this area is difficult to interpret.[44, 45] (See also Chapter 10.)

Implications for research and policy

The existence of socioeconomic differentials in cardiovascular disease risk provide an important model with which to study the basic causes of cardio-vascular disease. Attempts to explain the social patterning of cardiovascular disease should therefore advance our understanding of fundamental issues related to the aetiology and possible prevention of the disease.

The broad inequity within society is of primary importance in generating inequalities in cardiovascular disease risk. These inequalities cannot be simply reduced to behavioural and lifestyle differences between social groups. Furthermore, even where differences in smoking behaviour, dietary patterns and participation in physical activity are seen, they should not be considered as simply due to ignorance or fecklessness on the part of people living in materially less favoured circumstances. To take dietary practices as an example, those least able to purchase a healthy diet due to financial constraints are those most likely to be disadvantaged with regard to access to healthy micronutrient-dense food.

Over the recent period when inequalities in health have been widening, many indicators demonstrate increasing social polarisation. By 1993, one in three children in the UK lived in households with less than 50% of average UK income after housing costs; in 1979 this was less than 1 in 10.[46] Income inequalities have increased enormously over the same period. The income after deducting housing costs of the lowest decile group in 1991 was lower than the equivalent income of the lowest decile group in 1979.[47] This growth in income inequality has gone hand-in-hand with growth in socioeconomic inequalities in mortality,[47, 48] which includes widening inequalities in cardiovascular disease mortality.

The only economic argument in support of allowing income inequalities to widen is that the incentive of large income increases for the already wealthy in some way drives overall economic performance. This doctrine, strongly associated with the Thatcherite agenda of the 1980s, has recently been exploded. When labour productivity growth between 1979 and 1990 is plotted against income inequality in 1980, it is seen that, if anything, countries with lower levels of income inequality in 1980 had greater labour productivity growth over the following decade.[49] In 1979 the UK lay at around the average of the countries under consideration for both income inequality and labour productivity growth. Since then, inequality has massively increased in the UK, and the UK is now vying with the USA for the unfavourable title of 'most unequal country' in the industrialised world.

Tackling socioeconomic inequalities in cardiovascular disease risk involves addressing the processes leading to increasing social inequalities more generally and making firm decisions about what sort of society we would like to live in.

References

1   Drever F, Whitehead M. 1997. *Health Inequalities*. London: The Stationery Office.

2   Eachus J, Williams M, Chan P, Davey Smith G, Grainge M, Donovan J, Frankel S. 1996. Deprivation and cause-specific morbidity: Evidence from the Somerset and Avon survey of health. *British Medical Journal*; 312: 287–292.

3   Lynch J, Kaplan GA, Salonen R, Cohen RD, Salonen JT. 1995. Socioeconomic status and carotid atherosclerosis. *Circulation*; 92; 1786–1792.

4   Davey Smith G, Kuh D. Does early nutrition affect later health? Views from the 1930s and 1980s. In: Smith D (ed.) 1996. *The History of Nutrition in Britain in the Twentieth Century: Science, Scientists and Politics*. London: Routledge.

5   Kuh D, Davey Smith G. 1993. When is mortality risk determined? Historical insights into a current debate. *Social History of Medicine*; 6: 101–123.

6   Department of Health. 1995. *Variations in Health: What Can the Department of Health and the NHS Do?* London: Department of Health.

7   Davey Smith G, Hart C, Blane D, Hole D. 1998. Adverse socioeconomic conditions in childhood and cause-specific adult mortality: prospective observational study. *British Medical Journal*; 316: 1631–1635.

8   Davey Smith G, Hart C, Blane D, Gillis C, Hawthorne V. 1997. Socioeconomic position over the life course and mortality. *British Medical Journal*; 314: 547–552.

9   Jones HB. 1956. A special consideration of the ageing process, disease and life-expectancy. *Advances in Biology and Medical Physics*; 4: 281–337.

10 Alter R, Riley J. 1989. Frailty, sickness and death: Models of morbidity and mortality in historical populations. *Population Studies*; 43: 25–46.

11 Salhi M, Caselli G, Duchêne J, Egidi V, Santini A, Thiltgés E, Wunsch G. Assessing mortality differentials using life histories: a method and applications. In: Lopez A, Caselli G, Valkonen T (eds.) 1995. *Adult Mortality in Developed Countries: From Description to Explanation*. Oxford: Clarendon Press.

12 Mare RD. Socioeconomic careers and differential mortality among older men in the United States. In: Vallin J, D'Souza S, Palloni A (eds.) 1990. *Measurement and Analysis of Mortality: New Approaches*: 362–387. Oxford: Clarendon Press.

13 Valkonen T. 1987. Male mortality from ischaemic heart disease in Finland, in relation to region of birth and region of residence. *European Journal of Population*; 3: 61–83.

14 Koskinen S. 1994. *Origins of Regional Differences in Mortality from Ischaemic Heart Disease in Finland. National Research and Development Centre for Welfare and Health Research Report 41.* Helsinki: NAWH.

15 Blane D, Hart CL, Davey Smith G, Gillis CR, Hole DJ, Hawthorne VM. 1996. The association of cardiovascular disease risk factors with socioeconomic position during childhood and during adulthood. *British Medical Journal*; 313: 1434–1438.

16 Brunner EJ, Davey Smith G, Marmot M, Canner R, Beksinska M, O'Brien J. 1996. Childhood social circumstances and psychosocial and behavioural factors as determinants of plasma fibrinogen. *Lancet*; 347: 1008–1013.

17 Rimm EB, Ascherio A, Giovannucci E, Spiegelman D, Stampfer MJ, Willett WC. 1996. Vegetable, fruit, and cereal fiber intake and risk of coronary heart disease among men. *Journal of the American Medical Association*; 275: 447–451.

18 Lynch JW, Kaplan GA, Salonen JT. 1997. Why do poor people behave badly? Variation in adult health behaviours and psychosocial characteristics by stages of the socioeconomic lifecourse. *Social Science Medicine*; 44: 809–819.

19 Burnett JC. 1880. The prevention of hare-lip, cleft-palate, and other congenital defects: as also of hereditary disease and constitutional taints by the medicinal and nutritional treatment of their mother during pregnancy. *Homeopathic World*; 1880; Oct 1: 437–451.

20 Weiss S, Minot GR. Nutrition in relation to arteriosclerosis. In: Cowdry EV (ed.) 1933. *Arteriosclerosis: A Survey of the Problem*. New York: Macmillan Company.

21 Forsdahl A. 1977. Are poor living conditions in childhood and adolescents an important risk factor for arteriosclerotic heart disease? *British Journal of Preventive Social Medicine*; 31: 91–95.

22 Ben-Shlomo Y, Davey Smith G. 1991. Deprivation in infancy or in adult life: Which is more important for mortality risk? *Lancet*; 337: 530–534.

23 Barker DJP. Early nutrition and coronary heart disease. In: Davies DP (ed.) 1995. *Nutrition in Child Health*. London: Royal College of Physicians of London.

24 Rowett Research Institute. 1995. *Family Diet and Health in Pre-war Britain*. Dunfermline: Carnegie United Kingdom Trust, 1995.

25 Leitch I. 1951. Growth and health. *British Journal of Nutrition*; 5: 142–151.

26 Gunnell D, Davey Smith G, Frankel S, Nanchahal K, Braddon FEM, Pemberton J, Peters TJ. 1998. Childhood leg length and adult mortality – follow up of the Carnegie (Boyd Orr) Survey of diet and growth in pre-war Britain. *Journal of Epidemiology and Community Health*; 52; 3: 142–152.

27 Tannenbaum A. 1947. Effects of varying caloric intake upon tumor incidence and tumor growth. *Annals of New York Academy of Sciences*; 49: 5–18.

28 Albanes D, Jones, DY, Schatzkin A, Micozzi MS, Taylor PR. Adult stature and risk of cancer. 1988. *Cancer Research*; 48: 1658–1662.

29 Frankel SJ, Elwood P, Sweetnam P, Yarnell J, Davey Smith G. 1996. Birthweight, adult risk factors and incident coronary heart disease: The Caerphilly Study. *Public Health*; 110: 139–143.

30 Davey Smith G. Unpublished observations.

31 Leon J, Koupilova I, Lithell HI, Berglund L, Mohsen R, Vagero D et al. 1996. Failure to realise growth potential in utero and adult obesity in relation to blood pressure in 50 year old Swedish men. *British Medical Journal*; 312: 401–406.

32 Frankel S, Elwood P, Sweetnam P, Yarnell J, Davey Smith G. 1996. Birthweight, body-mass index in middle age, and incident coronary heart disease. *Lancet*; 348: 1478–1480.

33 Hertzman, C, Wiens M. 1996. Child development and long-term outcomes: a population health perspective and summary of successful interventions. *Social Science and Medicine*; 43: 1083–1095.

34 Davey Smith G, Hart C, Hole D, MacKinnon P, Gillis C, Watt G, Blane D, Hawthorne V. 1998. Education and occupational social class: which is the more important indicator of mortality risk? *Journal of Epidemiology and Community Health*; 52: 153–160.

35 Wadsworth M. 1996. Family and education as determinants of health. In: Blane D, Brunner E, Wilkinson R. *Health and Social Organisation*. London: Routledge.

36 Davey Smith G, Shipley MJ, Rose G. 1990. The magnitude and causes of socioeconomic differentials in mortality: further evidence from the Whitehall study. *Journal of Epidemiology and Community Health*; 44: 260–265.

37 Davey Smith G, Shipley MJ. 1991. Confounding of occupation and smoking: its magnitude and consequences. *Social Sciences Medicine*; 32: 1297–1300.

38 Davey Smith G, Bartley M, Blane D. 1994. Explanations for socioeconomic differentials in mortality: Evidence from Britain and elsewhere. *European Journal of Public Health*; 4: 131–144.

39 Davey Smith G, Wentworth D, Neaton JD, Stamler R, Stamler J. 1996. Socioeconomic differentials in mortality risk among men screened for the Multiple Risk Factor Intervention Trial: Part II – results for 20,224 black men. *American Journal of Public Health*; 86: 497–504.

40 Davey Smith G, Neaton JD, Wentworth D, Stamler R, Stamler J. 1996. Socioeconomic differentials in mortality risk among men screened for the Multiple Risk Factor Intervention Trial: Part I – results for 300,685 white men. *American Journal of Public Health*; 86: 486–496.

41 Marmot MG, Davey Smith G, Stansfeld S, Patel C, North F, Head J, White I, Brunner E, Feeney A. 1991. Inequalities in health twenty years on: The Whitehall II study of British civil servants. *Lancet*; 337: 1387–1394.

42 Brunner EJ, Marmot MG, White IR, O'Brien JR, Etherington MD, Slavin BM, Kearney EM, Davey Smith G. 1993. Gender and employment grade differences in blood cholesterol apolipoproteins and haemostatic factors in the Whitehall II study. *Atherosclerosis*; 102: 195–207.

43 Ferrie JE, Shipley MJ, Marmot MG, Stansfeld S, Davey Smith G. 1995. Health effects of anticipation of job change and non–employment: longitudinal data from the Whitehall II study. *British Medical Journal*; 311: 1264–1269.

44 Ferrie JE, Shipley MJ, Marmot MG, Stansfeld S, Davey Smith G. 1998. An uncertain future: The health effects of threats to employment security in white-collar men and women. *American Journal of Public Health*; 88: 1030–1036.

45 Carroll D, Davey Smith G, Bennet P. 1996. Some observations on health and socioeconomic status. *Journal of Health Psychology*; 1: 23–39.

46 Child Poverty Action Group. 1996. *Poverty: The Facts*. London: Child Poverty Action Group.

47 Davey Smith G, Egger M. 1993. Socioeconomic differentials in wealth and health. *British Medical Journal*; 307: 1085–1086.

48 McCarron P, Davey Smith G, Womersley JJ. 1994. Deprivation and mortality: Increasing differentials in Glasgow, 1979–1992. *British Medical Journal*; 309: 1481–1482.

49 Glynn and Miliband. 1994. *Paying for Inequality: The Economic Cost of Social Justice*. London: Rivers Oran Press.

50 Davey Smith G. 1997. Down at heart – the meaning and implications of social inequalities in cardiovascular disease. *Journal of the Royal College of Physicians of London*; 31: 414–424.

Acknowledgements

This chapter is an update based on the Lord Rayner Lecture 1996, given by Professor George Davey Smith at the Royal College of Physicians of London, and first published in the Journal of the Royal College of Physicians of London.[50]

Analysis of socioeconomic differentials in cardiovascular disease mortality in the Scottish Cohort was supported by a grant from the NHS Executive, Cardiovascular Disease and Stroke Research and Development Initiative. The author would like to thank Carole Hart for performing the analyses on the Scottish cohort and Debbie Tope, Anne Rennie and Adrian Field for help with preparation of the manuscript.

Chapter 4

The influence of income inequalities

Professor Richard Wilkinson

Trafford Centre for Medical Research, University of Sussex

Introduction

Income is an important determinant of the health status of individuals and populations. It seems that it is not so much a person's absolute level of income or standard of living which matters, as their income relative to others and the distribution of income across society as a whole.[1-4]

There is a strong tendency for people in economically more developed societies to have better health and longer life expectancies than people in less developed countries. However, the relationship between average living standards and average life expectancy becomes very much weaker among developed countries. Also, it appears that societies with smaller differences in incomes between rich and poor tend to achieve higher life expectancies, independently of the effect of the stage of economic development they have reached. The amount of income inequality is strongly correlated with national mortality rates and life expectancy: more egalitarian societies are healthier. Changes in income distribution over time also appear to be correlated with faster or slower rates of decline of mortality rates: in countries where there has been a widening income distribution, mortality rates tend to fall more slowly.

One possible explanation of these relationships is that, although improvements in people's absolute standard of living can bring about better health in poorer countries, they cease to do so in developed countries which have risen above a minimum standard of living associated with the 'epidemiological transition'. The epidemiological transition is the change from predominantly infectious causes of death, still common in poor countries, to the degenerative diseases, such as coronary heart disease, which have become the predominant cause of death in richer countries.[1]

However, *within* richer countries, there remains a strong gradient of health across income groups: higher income groups experience better health. This may be because income differences within countries parallel differences in social status which exerts a powerful influence on health. In other words, mortality *within* the developed countries is more influenced by relative rather than absolute income. This may be because income inequality acts as a measure of the burden of relative deprivation, which has an adverse effect on life expectancy in different societies.

Coronary heart disease is one of the most important causes of death in rich societies which have gone through the 'epidemiological transition' mentioned above. However, coronary heart disease mortality shows a strong social gradient in some but not all developed countries. Where it does show a strong social gradient, most of the gradient is apparently unexplained by behavioural and other risk factors.[5] In the UK, the social gradient in coronary heart disease mortality has increased dramatically, particularly during the period in which income differences have widened.[6] This chapter examines the relationship between coronary heart disease mortality and income distribution among the developed countries.

Coronary heart disease death rates and income distribution

Information on coronary heart disease death rates* and income distribution** were collected for eight countries: Australia, Canada, Italy, Luxembourg, Netherlands, Sweden, the UK and the United States, for 1986 or 1987 (the most recent data available when this study was undertaken). The income distribution for each of those countries was calculated as the percentage of total income received by the poorest 40%. Coronary heart disease death rates were then correlated with the income distribution. This cross-sectional analysis was carried out for six population groups: men and women separately in the three age groups 45–54, 55–64, and 65–74 years.

The results show an inverse relationship between the coronary heart disease death rate and equitable income distribution: mortality tended to be lower in more egalitarian countries (see Figures 1 and 2 for ages 45–54, Figures 3 and 4 for ages 55–64 and Figures 5 and 6 for ages 65–74). The strongest association was found among women aged 45–54 (see Figure 2). This was the only group in which the association between coronary heart disease death rates and income distribution was statistically significant. However, given that there were only eight countries in each of the analyses, relationships would have to be very strong to reach statistical significance.

---

*   Coronary heart disease mortality rates were taken from the World Health Organization's *World Health Statistics* for the same countries and years as those for which the income distribution statistics were available.

**   Data on income distribution (prepared for a previous study – see reference 7) are available for all those OECD countries for which the Luxembourg Income Study's data bank has internationally comparable data on income distribution. Income was defined as personal disposable income (after taxes and benefits) for households and was adjusted for household size.

In each age group, the associations between income inequality and coronary heart disease mortality were stronger among women than among men, and in both sexes the relationships became successively weaker in older age groups and was non-existent among men aged 65–74 years.

In most of these groups, mortality rates for Italy and the UK were off the trend: for Italy they were much lower than expected and for the UK much higher than expected.

Figure 1 *Coronary heart disease death rate for men aged 45–54 years in relation to income distribution, 1986–1987*

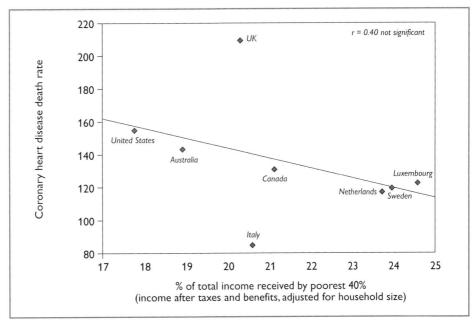

Figure 2 *Coronary heart disease death rate for women aged 45–54 years in relation to income distribution, 1986–1987*

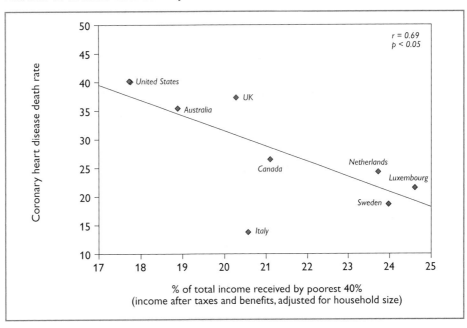

Figure 3   Coronary heart disease death rate for men aged 55–64 years in relation to income distribution, 1986–1987

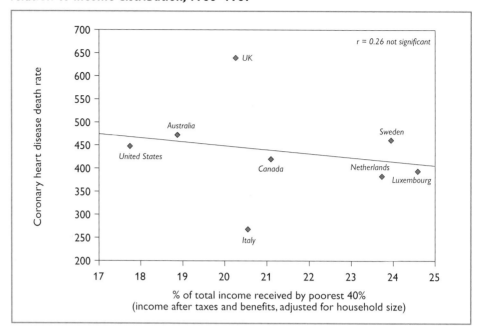

Figure 4   Coronary heart disease death rate for women aged 55–64 years in relation to income distribution, 1986–1987

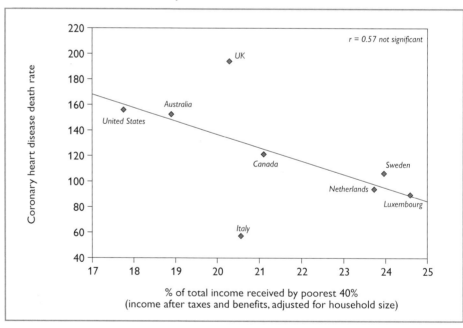

Figure 5 Coronary heart disease death rate for men aged 65–74 years in relation to income distribution, 1986–1987

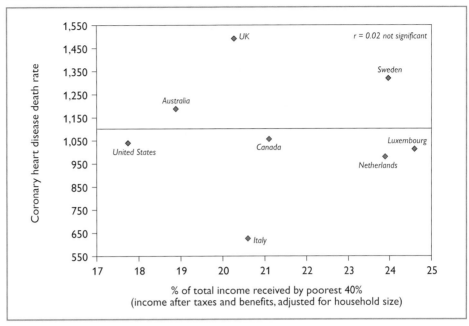

Figure 6 Coronary heart disease death rate for women aged 65–74 years in relation to income distribution, 1986–1987

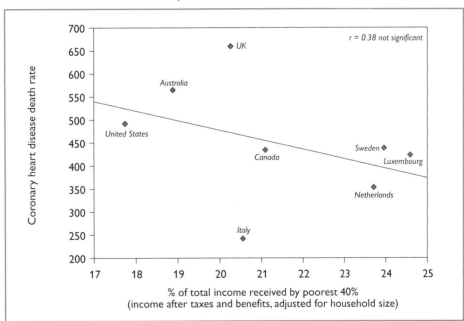

Do coronary heart disease death rates fall more slowly in countries where income differences have widened?

It is also interesting to examine whether countries which have experienced a reduction in income differences over time also experience a faster rate of decline in coronary heart disease mortality. In order to do this, information on *changes* in income distribution over a period of time (at least five years) were calculated for five countries: Canada, France, Sweden, the UK and the United States (see footnote* on page 52).

Figure 7 *Annual change in coronary heart disease death rate of men aged 45–54 years in relation to change in income distribution*

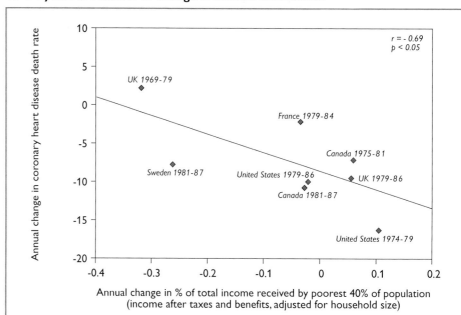

Figure 8 *Annual change in coronary heart disease death rate of women aged 45–54 years in relation to change in income distribution*

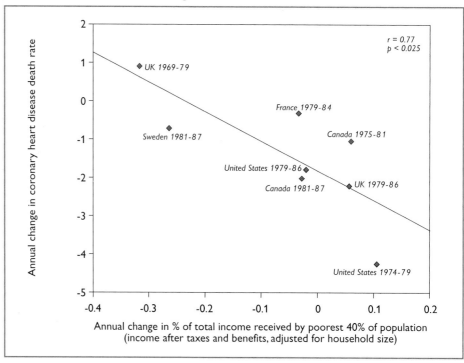

It was found that countries which had experienced a *reduction* in income differences over time also experienced a faster rate of decline in coronary heart disease mortality. A reduction in the scale of income differences was associated with a faster rate of decline in coronary heart disease mortality in both men and women in all three age groups (see Figures 7–12). This correlation was strongest in the 45–54 year age group, for both men and women. The correlation was also seen for both sexes in the 55–64 year age group but was lower in the oldest age group. Although the relationship weakened in the older age groups as it did in the cross-sectional analyses (see Figures 1–6), unlike in the cross-sectional analyses there was no consistent difference between the sexes in the strength of the relationship.

Figure 9 *Annual change in coronary heart disease death rate of men aged 55–64 years in relation to change in income distribution*

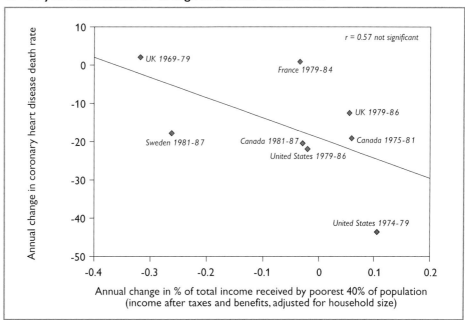

Figure 10 *Annual change in coronary heart disease death rate of women aged 55–64 years in relation to change in income distribution*

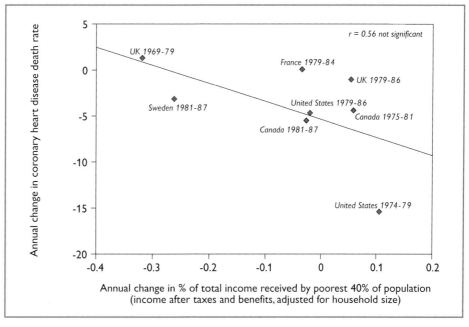

Figure 11 *Annual change in coronary heart disease death rate of men aged 65–74 years in relation to change in income distribution*

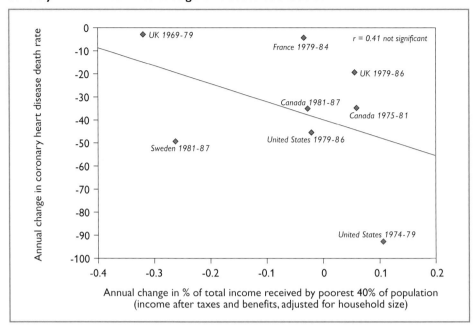

Figure 12 *Annual change in coronary heart disease death rate of women aged 65–74 years in relation to change in income distribution*

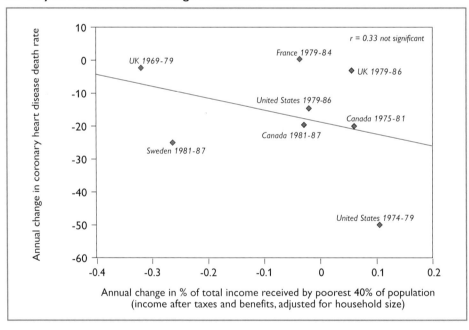

---

    *   Data were collected for those countries for which it was possible to identify two years of data, between five and ten years apart, which would enable rates of change to be calculated. For Sweden and France there were two data points at least five years apart, and for Canada, the UK and the United States there were three years of data, allowing estimates of change over two periods. For some countries data were available for only one year, preventing any analysis of change for those countries. Data on changes in income distribution over time were therefore calculated for: Canada 1975–81 and 1981–87; France 1979–84; Sweden 1981–87; UK 1969–79 and 1979–86; and the United States 1974–79 and 1979–86.

In the cross-sectional analysis, age-specific mortality rates were correlated with the income distribution data. As the data on changes over time covered periods of different length, the changes in income distribution and mortality were expressed as annual rates of change.

What is the explanation?

Both the cross-sectional analysis (see Figures 1–6) and the analysis of changes over time (see Figures 7–12) suggest that coronary heart disease mortality is associated with income distribution. Countries with a more equitable income distribution seem to have a lower mortality from coronary heart disease. Countries which have become more egalitarian seem to experience a faster rate of decline in coronary heart disease mortality. These observations are particularly marked among the younger age groups.

The explanation for these relationships is far from clear. Income inequality is measured across all age groups, regardless of whether the relatively poor are young or old. It is not possible to tell from the data presented in this chapter:

–   whether any relationship between income distribution within a society and coronary heart disease mortality springs directly from an association between individual mortality and the relative incomes of those individuals, or

–   whether people's mortality is also affected by whether they live in a more or less egalitarian society, regardless of their own relative incomes.

Given that higher mortality rates, within many societies, are found among those with lower income, it seems more likely that most of the effect of inequality results from the influence of low relative income on the mortality rates of the relatively poor themselves – not from any wider societal effects.

However, even if this were so, the reasons why the effect is less pronounced among older people are unclear. It may be because mortality among older people is affected less by relative income, or because the international differences in the burden of low relative income fall less on older people than on the rest of the population. It is possible that coronary heart disease among older people may be just as sensitive to changes in their socioeconomic status, but that their relative incomes varied less from one country to another and from one period to the next than did the relative incomes of younger people. This might be the case if income distribution were affected by changes in earnings among people of working age. Whatever the explanation, the pattern is a familiar one: although inequalities in mortality continue into old age, their magnitude is usually smaller in older age than among people in their 30s, 40s and 50s.

How low social status may affect coronary heart disease

The extent of income inequality may well be serving as an indicator of how hierarchical the social hierarchy of a society is. Wider income differences would then indicate a heavier burden of relative deprivation on its mortality rates. In a more egalitarian society, perhaps most people experience themselves as part of the main body of society, as more or less the social equals of others. In less egalitarian societies it may be that more people will be aware of social differences, of inferiority or superiority, of failure and exclusion, of low social status and loss of self-esteem.

The work of Shively on captive macaque monkeys has demonstrated that low social status affects a number of coronary risk factors. Among captive animals whose social status could be manipulated and whose diet and environment controlled, Shively found that low status animals developed atherosclerosis more quickly, had a poorer blood lipid profile, higher blood pressure and an increased tendency to central obesity[8,9] (a type of obesity particularly associated with higher risk of coronary heart disease).

These effects were associated with the chronic stress experienced by low status animals. Shively says "current subordinates received more aggression, engaged in less affiliation, and spent more time alone than dominants. Furthermore, they spent more time fearfully scanning the social environment and displayed more behavioural depression than dominants."[10]

This picture is very compatible with Sapolsky's findings of the effects of social status among wild baboons.[11] He too sees the process as starting with the chronic stress caused by low social status, which then causes elevated cortisol levels which can lead to a suppression of blood lipids which are protective against coronary heart disease. Similarly, after pointing out that it is known that sustained glucocorticoid over-exposure can adversely affect blood lipid profiles, Sapolsky says he found that sustained social subordinance among baboons was associated with these and other adverse circulatory changes.

Low status civil servants within the Whitehall Study were found to have higher rates of fibrinogen which, as well as being responsive to immediate stress and an important risk factor for heart disease, may well be affected by chronic stress.[12] Brunner has discussed the similarities between some of the biological effects of social status among humans and non-human primates.[13]

In addition, the emphasis placed here on relative income and on social position - rather than on the direct effects of absolute material circumstances – accords well with the research which has pointed to the importance of psychosocial factors in health and in the generation of health inequalities.[14-20] Among these are: sense of control, social support and social affiliation, life events, and job insecurity, all of which may be seen as impacting on levels of chronic stress. (See Chapter 10.)

Policy implications

Most multi-factorial intervention studies report limited success in reducing rates of coronary heart disease and fewer still describe strategies which are effective in reducing the social inequalities in heart disease.[21-23] The conclusion that should perhaps be drawn is that the kinds of factors which health care workers, community development workers and researchers are able to manipulate at the local and personal level may not be the crucial ones. If so, then the question is: would a greater impact be achieved by addressing those factors associated with relative deprivation and the degree of inequality in society which are potentially manipulable at a societal level, whether by governments or as part of a wider process of social and economic change?

When addressing health inequalities it is important to establish the relationship between inequalities in mortality and overall national mortality rates. Does the increased burden of illness associated with deprivation contribute to higher national mortality rates, or is their effect offset by a tendency for mortality rates higher up the social scale to be lower than they would have been had relative deprivation been reduced? In other words, are health inequalities simply an issue of social justice and the distribution of a given amount of disease in society, or are health inequalities also a reflection of a net increase in the burden of unnecessary illness? If the relationship between national mortality rates and income inequality reflects, as seems most likely, the scale of the burden of relative deprivation in society, greater health inequalities are likely to contribute to higher overall mortality levels. Effective policies to tackle them may then be one of the best ways of improving national mortality rates.

The scale of income inequality in the UK widened more rapidly during the 1980s than it did in any other developed market economy[24] and the UK's relative position in the international league table for life expectancy slipped, despite national and local health promotion activity. As the health effects of government economic and fiscal policies may have a greater impact on health status than most of the interventions that health professionals can manipulate, it is essential that government strategy takes this into account.

Conclusion

The data presented in this chapter suggest that national premature mortality rates from coronary heart disease in different countries are higher in countries where income differences are greater, and have been falling more slowly in countries where income differences have widened. The relationship between income distribution within the whole population and age-specific coronary heart disease mortality rates is weaker at older than at younger ages when comparing countries within the same time frame and when looking at change over periods of five to ten years.

References

1   Wilkinson RG. 1996. *Unhealthy Societies: The Afflictions of Inequality*. London: Routledge.

2   Kaplan GA, Pamuk E, Lynch JW, Cohen RD, Balfour JL. 1996. Inequality in income and mortality in the United States: analysis of mortality and potential pathways. *British Medical Journal*; 312: 999–1003.

3   Kawachi I, Kennedy BP. 1997. The relationship of income inequality to mortality – does the choice of indicator matter? *Social Science and Medicine*; 45 (7): 1121–1128.

4   Wilkinson RG. 1997. Health inequalities: relative or absolute material standards? *British Medical Journal*; 314: 591–595.

5   Marmot MG, Rose G, Shipley M, Hamilton PJS. 1978. Employment grade and coronary heart disease in British civil servants. *Journal of Epidemiology and Community Health*; 32: 244–249.

6   Drever F, Whitehead M, Roden M. 1996. Current patterns and trends in male mortality by social class (based on occupation). *Population Trends*; 86: 15–20.

7   Wilkinson RG. 1993. Income and health. In: *Health, Wealth and Poverty. Medical World*, special edition.

8   Shively CA, Clarkson TB. 1994. Social status and coronary artery atherosclerosis in female monkeys. *Arteriosclerosis and Thrombosis*; 14: 721–726.

9   Kaplan JR, Adams MR, Clarkson TB, Manuck SB, Shively CA, Williams JK. 1996. Psychosocial factors, sex-differences, and atherosclerosis – lessons from animal-models. *Psychosomatic Medicine*; 58 (6): 598–611.

10   Shively CA, Laird KL, Anton RF. 1997. The behavior and physiology of social stress and depression in female cynomolgus monkeys. *Biological Psychiatry*; 41: 871–882.

11   Sapolsky RM. 1993. Endocrinology alfresco: psychoendocrine studies of wild baboons. *Recent Progress in Hormone Research*; 48: 437–468.

12 Brunner, E. 1996. Childhood social circumstances and psychosocial and behavioural factors as determinants of plasma fibrinogen. *Lancet*; 347: 1008–1013.

13 Brunner E. 1997. Stress and the biology of inequality. *British Medical Journal*; 314: 1472–1476.

14 Ferrie JE, Shipley MJ, Marmot MG, Stansfeld S, Davey Smith G. 1995. Health effects of anticipation of job change and non-employment: longitudinal data from the Whitehall II study. *British Medical Journal*; 311: 1264–1269.

15 Berkman LF. 1995. The role of social relations in health promotion. *Psychosomatic Research*; 57: 245–254.

16 Berkman LF, Syme SL. 1979. Social networks, host resistance and mortality: a nine year follow up study of Alameda County residents. *American Journal of Epidemiology*; 109: 186.

17 Bosma H, Marmot MG, Hemingway H, Nicholson A, Brunner EJ, Stansfeld S. 1997. Low job control and risk of coronary heart disease in the Whitehall II study. *British Medical Journal*; 314: 558–565.

18 Rosengren A, Orth-Gomer K, Wedel H, Wilhelmsen L. 1993. Stressful life events, social support, and mortality in men born in 1933. *British Medical Journal*; 307: 1102–1105.

19 Siegrist J, Peter R, Junge A, Cremer P, Seidel D. 1990. Low status control, high effort at work and coronary heart disease: prospective evidence from blue-collar men. *Social Science and Medicine*; 31: 1127–1134.

20 Lovallo WR. 1997. *Stress and Health: Biological and Psychological Interactions*. London: Sage.

21 Multiple Risk Factor Intervention Trial Group. 1982. The Multiple Intervention Risk Factor Intervention Trial – risk factor changes and mortality results. *Journal of the American Medical Association*; 248: 1465–1476.

22 Syme SL. To prevent disease: the need for a new approach. In: Blane D, Brunner E, Wilkinson RG (eds.) 1996. *Health and Social Organization*. London: Routledge.

23 Ebrahim S, Davey Smith G. 1997. Systematic review of randomised controlled trials of multiple risk factor interventions for preventing coronary heart disease. *British Medical Journal*; 314: 1666–1674.

24 Hills J. 1995. *Inquiry into Income and Wealth. Volume 2*. York: Joseph Rowntree Foundation.

Acknowledgements

This chapter is by Professor Richard Wilkinson of the Trafford Centre for Medical Research, University of Sussex and the International Centre for Health and Society at University College London. Financial support from the Paul Hamlyn Foundation is gratefully acknowledged.

Chapter 5

Material circumstances: possibilities for local action

Dr Andrew Lyon

Forward Scotland*

Introduction

Scotland has the fourth highest all cause death rate for men and the second highest for women of 27 major industrialised countries. Glasgow's death rates are 11% higher than the national average for Scotland, and death rates for those aged under 65 are 35% higher.[1]

The most striking feature of health in Glasgow is the variation in health between affluent and deprived areas. This difference is largely caused by the increased vulnerability to ill health and the lack of well-being which poverty brings in its wake, rather than by specific causes of death. The tendency to premature death outweighs any specific hazard other than cigarette smoking, which is itself related to poverty. Of the 6,700 deaths among the under-65s which occur each year in Glasgow, 2,600 are associated with this difference in health between the rich and the poor.[2]

Health promotion aimed at changing individual behaviour is not enough. People's health behaviour interacts with the social conditions and the environment in which they live. For example, in a survey of 160 households in the Drumchapel area of Glasgow, 75% of adults smoked, and 70% wanted to give up but said they would not bother trying because they felt that they would fail.[3]

This chapter looks at how local organisations in and around Glasgow have joined together to tackle poverty and unemployment through policy development and related action programmes. It examines Glasgow's state of health and outlines some of the ways in which these problems are being tackled and the underlying rationale for the activity.

---

* Dr Andrew Lyon is Development Manager at Forward Scotland, a Glasgow-based charity responsible for sustainable development in Scotland. Until 1996 he was Coordinator of the Glasgow Healthy City Project.

Glasgow's state of health

Major causes of death in Glasgow

There are approximately 13,200 deaths in Glasgow each year. Nearly 80% of all deaths are attributed to four major causes: respiratory diseases (excluding cancers), cancers, coronary heart disease and strokes.

The total premature death rate for Glasgow is some 35% higher than the rate for Scotland as a whole. The death rate from coronary heart disease in Glasgow is almost 40% higher than the average for Scotland, for lung cancer about 50% higher, and for respiratory disease about 80% higher (see Figure 1).

Figure 1   Major causes of premature death (under 65 years), Glasgow City, 1993

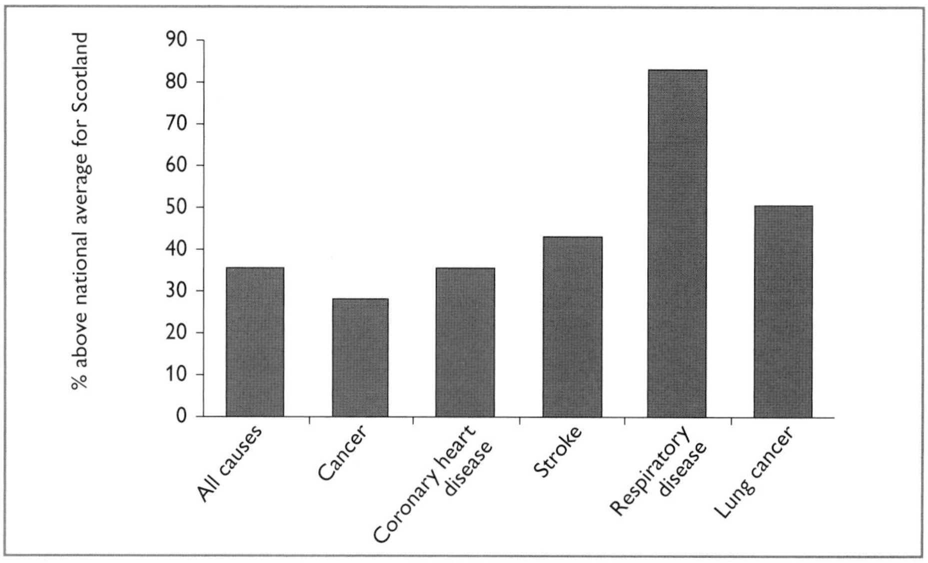

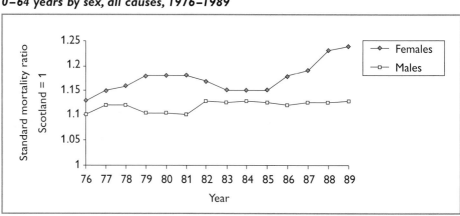

Source: See reference 4.

Although from the 1970s onwards there has been a downward trend in death rates for all causes among people up to the age of 64 years, Glasgow is improving more slowly than the rest of Scotland. This means that the gap between Glasgow's premature mortality and that of the whole of Scotland is becoming greater. While the rates for both men and women are becoming worse, the rate for women relative to men is worsening more quickly, as illustrated by the widening gap from 1984 onwards (see Figure 2).

Figure 2   Standardised mortality ratios for Greater Glasgow Health Board, 0–64 years by sex, all causes, 1976–1989

Source: See reference 4.

Of the 13,200 deaths each year in Glasgow, it is estimated that at least 2,000 could be prevented if the appropriate remedial action was taken early enough.[2]

Major causes of ill health in Glasgow
Relatively little is known about the level of morbidity (ill health) in the general population since routine data are not collected until patients attend hospital. Inpatient admission data, supplemented with information from community health services, show that over a quarter of hospital beds for patients resident in the Greater Glasgow Health Board area are used by patients with heart and circulatory diseases or stroke.[4]

The best of health and the worst of health

Health is not evenly distributed across the city. The health status of Glaswegians varies geographically, socioeconomically and by gender. Men living in the more deprived areas are three times more likely to die prematurely (before their 65th birthday) than their more affluent counterparts. Women living in the poorest areas are twice as likely to die prematurely than their more affluent neighbours.

Income and wealth are not evenly distributed across the city. It is indisputable that those who live in the most deprived areas of the city have much poorer health, regardless of how this is measured, than those who live in the more affluent areas.

To facilitate analysis of these differences, the Greater Glasgow Health Board has devised eight 'neighbourhood types' covering the city. Neighbourhood types 1 and 2 are those with the most affluent socioeconomic profiles, while types 7 and 8 are the most socioeconomically deprived. The differences in neighbourhood types for five main indicators are set out in Figure 3.

Figure 3   *Glasgow City household characteristics: comparison of household types*

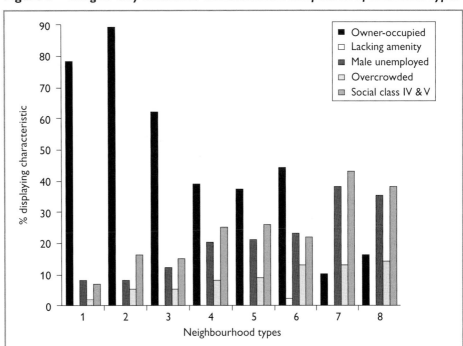

Source: See reference 4.

There is a very strong positive association between disadvantage and mortality; premature mortality was more than twice as high in neighbourhood types 7 and 8 compared with types 1 and 2 in 1981 and 1989 (see Figure 4).

Figure 4 *Standardised mortality ratios for neighbourhood types in Glasgow City, age 0–64 years, both sexes, 1981 and 1989*

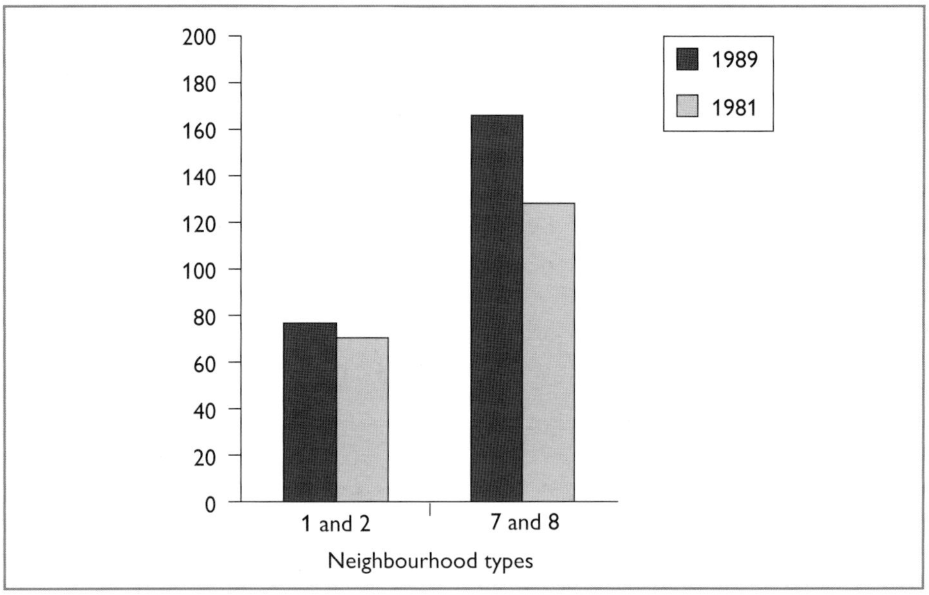

Source: See reference 4.

The same pattern is seen for individual causes of mortality, thus giving weight to the 'susceptibility to risk' argument, that the poor are more susceptible to illness for any given level of exposure or risk. Morbidity shows the same pattern again, as can be seen from data on hospital discharge rates for acute specialities (see Figure 5).

Figure 5 *Standardised hospital discharge rates (acute specialities) for neighbourhood types, age 0–64, both sexes, 1981 and 1989*

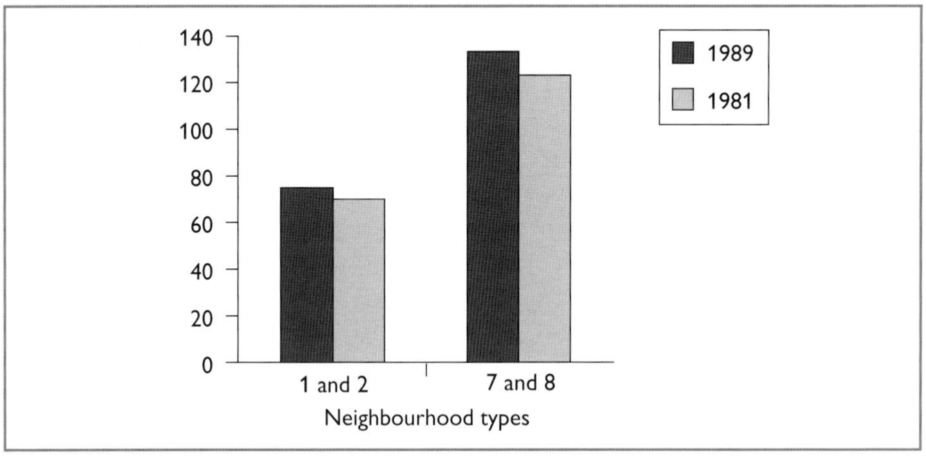

Source: See reference 4.

Factors involved in the relationship between poverty and ill health

The relationship between poverty and ill health is now widely accepted in Glasgow, against a wider background of research relating to health inequalities and income in the UK. It is worth examining some of the main factors implicated in these differences since they have great bearing on the actions which must be taken in Glasgow in aiming to eradicate these differences.

One explanation of poor health is that it is simply the outcome of individual differences in behaviour. However, behaviour is heavily influenced by social and economic circumstances.[5] If these circumstances are improved then, firstly, they will in themselves lead to better health. Secondly, they will encourage and enable more people to adopt health-enhancing behaviour.

Income

Income has one of the strongest influences on health. It influences where people live, the type of house people live in, access to leisure and space, education, diet, clothing and fuel.

In Glasgow a large proportion of people have an inadequate income.[6] The average official rate of unemployment in the city as a whole is 15%. Unofficial estimates suggest 25%. This rises to over 40% in some disadvantaged areas. Unemployment is also implicated in higher rates of mental illness, early death and suicide. In most of the city's disadvantaged areas over 60% of households are in receipt of housing benefit, and 75% of children receive clothing grants and free school meals. This implies that some families are living in poverty through being in low-paid employment. By contrast, in the wealthier Glasgow suburbs of Bearsden and Milngavie, where a low percentage of people receive housing benefit, only 8% of children receive footwear or clothing grants.[6] Economic initiatives, aimed at producing more fairly-paid jobs in the city, need to be an integral part of planning for health.

Housing

Housing and the housing environment also have a considerable impact on health, since most people spend most of their time in and around their homes. The poor condition of Glasgow's housing stock was again highlighted in the 1991 *Housing Condition Survey*[7] which indicated that 104,000 homes in the city show signs of dampness and condensation. Half of these were in the public sector. Damp and cold housing is more likely to be occupied by those in poverty, a circumstance which creates a vicious circle, since heating costs for such households are prohibitively high. Damp and cold housing in Glasgow has been shown to have a direct effect on respiratory infection, tiredness and fever, particularly among children. An associated effect, which has not been measured, is the impact on life chances which comes from days of missed schooling through illness associated with damp housing and poverty. Despite dramatic improvements in housing, the 1991 census identified that 40% of households in the peripheral estates had population densities of more than one per room, compared to 4% of households in more affluent areas.

It is also worth noting that mortality rates in winter are 15%–20% higher than those in summer. The most likely explanation for this is the change in the ambient air temperature inside the home. Elderly people and those on a low income are most at risk. The imposition of tax on domestic fuel bills is likely to have made this situation worse.

While great strides have been made in housing improvement in Glasgow, there is still poor housing stock which is associated with poor health. The relative effect of housing improvement on health compared to improvements in a range of social and economic improvements including housing, remains unknown. More research is needed.

The local residential environment also has an impact on health; both its condition and the amenities which it offers are likely to have an impact on health as well as air- and water-borne pollution, noise, and safety from accidents, crime and the fear of crime.

Transport

The movement of goods and people can both promote and damage health. Transport can damage health, principally through accidents, pollution, noise, vibration, stress and anxiety. However, transport enables access to the amenities which contribute to normal inclusion in the everyday life of the city. Using shops, getting to work, travelling to leisure facilities, and visiting friends and family are essential aspects of everyday life for which transport is often necessary. However, access to transport is not evenly distributed across the population. Glasgow's deprived areas have very low rates of car ownership compared to other areas in Scotland or the UK, highlighting the need for good public transport for those who experience poverty.

Health services

Health services play an important part in the early identification of disease and illness through primary prevention work and screening services. When illness exists, access to good quality local health care is an important contributory factor in recovery. It has been argued that an inverse care law exists in the provision of medical services: that is, that medical services are not located or provided where the need is greatest.

Control

In addition to the material effects of deprivation upon health, there is growing evidence that a sense of control over life, a sense of belonging and a feeling of being a net contributor to life have a strong influence on well-being. Studies in the United States[8] and Canada[9] suggest that those with a wide circle of friends and social contacts experience less illness and have a greater chance of recovery should they become ill. Poverty and its associated difficulties are associated with mental health problems and are stress-inducing. Not being able to pay bills, incurring debts, damp housing and poor living conditions lead to a feeling of low control over life, which in turn may lead to poor health outcomes. The effectiveness of any action taken to improve health in the city will therefore be greater if more residents are involved in decisions which affect their lives.

The principles guiding local action in Glasgow

Action to address these problems in Glasgow has been guided by four key principles:

- The poor in Glasgow are more vulnerable to overall morbidity and mortality. Coronary heart disease itself makes little difference to the length and quality of life of these people: if coronary heart disease were eradicated, people would most likely die of some other cause at the same age in the same circumstances. The important issue is people's susceptibility to disease and death.

- Health is created by everyday life and not by the health care sector. As it is created by human actions, it is therefore amenable to change.

- No single organisation, group, political party or any other grouping on its own can produce health.

- Local participation is effective, and Glasgow has a strong tradition of participation.

Policy areas

To have sustainable healthy cities, three areas must be nurtured: economic vitality, environmental integrity and social well-being (see Figure 6). As actions across spheres are integrated, more health is created. If actions are pursued separately, health is undermined.

Figure 6   *A model for sustainable healthy cities*

Economic vitality

Environmental integrity

Sustainable

Equitable   Liveable

Health and well-being

Social well-being

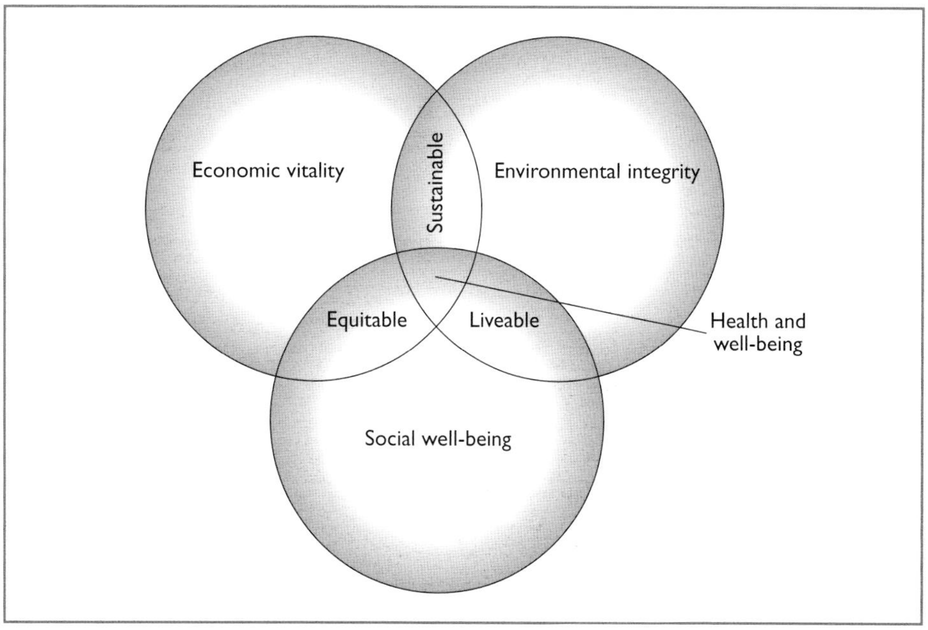

Source: See reference 10.

The basis for local action

This approach points to four principles for local action:

- *Partnership*
  Partnership is an essential principle given that the responsibility for health is very wide.

- *Policy integration and a balance between economic, social and environmental spheres of activity*
  No one sphere can be pursued indefinitely without damaging aspects of the other spheres. The aim is that economic policies should not compromise social or environmental objectives.

- *Local participation at various levels*

- *Fairness*
  Policies must be redistributive across a wide range of socioeconomic groups and across the life cycle.

Examples of local action in Glasgow

Glasgow has several local initiatives which adopt the principles above. Three examples are:

– the Glasgow Regeneration Alliance

– the Strathclyde Regional Council Social Strategy, and

– the Glasgow Healthy City Project.

These are described below. There have been concerted attempts to evaluate these initiatives, but it is difficult to raise funds for evaluation. Earmarked money for a national evaluation strategy, to review the effectiveness of projects such as those taking place in Glasgow, would be very useful.

The Glasgow Regeneration Alliance

The Glasgow Regeneration Alliance initiative is a partnership of Glasgow City Council, Strathclyde Regional Council, the Glasgow Development Agency and Scottish Homes. The term 'partnership' conceals the many difficult negotiations that have to take place before organisations, with quite different aims, can agree on joint objectives.

The document produced by these negotiations, the Glasgow Regeneration Alliance Strategy,[11] agrees an integrated and coordinated investment strategy in the eight most deprived areas of the city with respect to unemployment and numbers of people on housing benefit. It covers areas such as: industrial business development, community involvement, housing development, shopping and leisure facilities, and infrastructure and environment. Although health care was originally omitted from the document, it was later included and the Glasgow Health Board is now a full partner in the strategy.

Strathclyde Regional Council Social Strategy

With the *Strathclyde Regional Council Social Strategy*,[12] mainstream resources are focused on reducing disadvantage and building stronger communities, with the aim of improving quality of life. The strategy covers 12 areas including deprivation, urban regeneration, community empowerment, education, transport, and safety. It gives proposals for action in relation to each area.

Strathclyde has a good track record for community involvement and has recently further decentralised decision-making so that whole communities can get more involved in how their money is spent. With the demise of the Regional Councils in Scotland in the mid-1990s, this strategy has been reformulated by the new City Council.

Glasgow Healthy City Project

The Glasgow Healthy City Project[1] is a partnership between statutory and voluntary agencies, academic and health care organisations. It aims to formulate policies which influence health in the city. Senior level staff from these organisations are involved so that they are able to deliver their commitment to the project in terms of resources. The city's three main statutory organisations have all committed resources. The project, which started with a small number of staff in 1989, now receives in the region of £5 million funding and involves

350–400 workers, either directly or as part of their duties and responsibilities at the local level around specific projects and programmes.

Policy development work

The Glasgow Healthy City Project has devised a health plan for the whole city. The housing department now has a strategy which explicitly sets out to improve health by investing in housing. The plan addresses deprivation, housing, health, ethnic minorities and issues raised by the 1991 census. Local versions of the plan have now been produced.

Local action programme

The local action programme aims to value local experience and ask people what difference the City's commitment to the Healthy City Project has made for people who live in areas of great need.

Information and training

In addition to local conferences and seminars, Healthy City Project workers participate in international conferences, teach on undergraduate and postgraduate courses, and help with the production of materials in ethnic minority languages. The project also undertakes, jointly with directors of public health, local consultation projects in which people are asked what their health needs are and what is needed to improve their health. These needs and proposals are then developed into a sustainable strategy.

National and international liaison

The Glasgow Healthy City project team has worked with the Organisation for European Cooperation and Development on a pilot project called the Ecological City Project and with the European Union to explore the implications, for public health in Glasgow, of Article 129 of the Maastricht Treaty and Article 152 of the Amsterdam Treaty. This programme will systematically follow the council's capital investment programme for housing. Comprehensive social surveys and physical surveys of indoor air quality will be conducted in several hundred households before and after capital improvement. Early indications are that modest housing investment reaps significant reductions in health care use, even within the first year after renovation.

Glasgow Action for Warm Houses project

One quarter of the city's council tenants cannot afford to pay their fuel bills. The aim of the Glasgow Action for Warm Houses project, a partnership between City Housing and the fuel boards, is to reduce the proportion of disposable income spent on fuel to no more than 10%. Activities to achieve this include: an energy audit of all housing in the city, energy efficiency measures, capital investment, and alterations to fuel tariff structures such as standing charges, which currently disadvantage those on low incomes.

Capital investment in upgrading housing stock is not the solution for small households. Even with the best housing stock possible, many residents would still not have the income to pay their fuel bills because they are simply too poor. Also, the investment needed to improve Glasgow's housing stock is not currently available.

Local action to address food and poverty

Thirty per cent of people in the most deprived areas of Glasgow seldom eat fruit and vegetables. However, there are no differences in the consumption of skimmed milk or in consumption of fat between the least and most deprived areas. This suggests that differences in cost and availability between the most and least deprived areas are important in explaining health behaviour.

A Joint Working Group was set up to address food supply problems. The group includes representatives of the Strathclyde Poverty Alliance, the Healthy City Project and a range of people from both the private and public sector. It is recognised that the problems of food availability and cost are related to what happens at an international level, and that action needs to be taken to increase the supply of affordable food throughout Strathclyde. A survey of several different communities has been carried out to define the barriers to the consumption of wholesome food and find ways of effectively tackling them.

A study conducted in the East End of the City aimed to improve consumers' knowledge of healthy eating and cooking skills but was not successful. The consumption of fruit and vegetables increased by only 4%–5%. The researchers concluded that action for healthy eating should be aimed at the retailer, the wholesaler and the producer rather than at the consumer.

Another aspect of the food and poverty strategy is the establishment of food co-operatives, alternative marketing strategies and electronic networks. Food co-operatives are not a substitute for local shops. If the food co-op fails, or where resistance to co-ops is high, then local consumers are dependent on private sector shops. Local shops also have to be encouraged to provide a reasonable range of wholesome food at prices which people can afford. In some cases the service provided to local people is extremely poor with cartels on price operating among shopkeepers.

Electronic networks may support local shops in providing a better service by connecting them to a centrally based supply depot. This would encourage guaranteed delivery for a wider range of goods, lessen cash flow problems, and increase the turnover for local shopkeepers. In doing so, consumers could benefit from a wider range of affordable foods and other goods.

Figure 7   *The legend of Sisyphus*

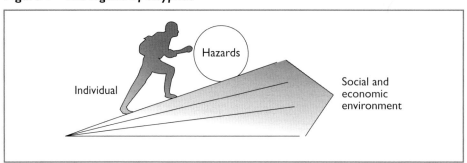

Conclusion

Figure 7 shows Sisyphus pushing the boulder of hazards up the hill of social and economic disadvantage. A conventional intervention would focus on the size of the boulder, or would aim to make Sisyphus stronger by getting him to stop smoking. The unconventional approach as adopted by the projects described above, is to tackle the slope of the hill, as well as the size of the boulder and the strength of the individual.

References

1   Lyon A. 1995. *Working Together for Glasgow's Health: The Glasgow City Health Plan 1995*. Glasgow: Glasgow Healthy City Project.

2   Forwell G. 1993. *Director of Public Health Annual Report*. Glasgow: Greater Glasgow Health Board.

3   Kennedy A. 1993. *Local Voices, Local Lives: The Story of the Kendoon Community Health Profile*. Glasgow: Drumchapel Community Health Project.

4   Greater Glasgow Health Board. 1992. *Director of Public Health, Annual Report 1992*. Glasgow: Greater Glasgow Health Board.

5   Watt GCM, Ecob R. 1992. Mortality in Glasgow and Edinburgh: a paradigm of inequality and health. *Journal of Epidemiology and Community Health*; 46; 498-505.

6   Economic Development Department. 1993. *Glasgow City Council Quarterly Economic Bulletin*. Glasgow: Glasgow City Council.

7   Glasgow City Housing. 1991. *The Housing Condition Survey*. Glasgow: Glasgow City Council.

8   Berkman L, Syme SL. 1979. Social networks, host resistance and mortality: A nine-year follow-up study of Alameda county residents. *American Journal of Epidemiology*; 109; 2: 186-204.

9   Canadian Institute for Advanced Research. 1991. *Publication No. 5. The Determinants of Health*. Toronto: Canadian Institute for Advanced Research.

10   Developed from an idea by Trevor Hancock.

11   Glasgow Regeneration Alliance. 1993. *Shaping the Future: A Commitment to Area Regeneration*. Glasgow: Glasgow Regeneration Alliance.

12   *Strathclyde Regional Council Social Strategy 1993*. Glasgow: Strathclyde Regional Council.

Chapter 6

Interventions to tackle social inequalities in coronary heart disease: what works?

Professor Dr Louise Gunning-Schepers

Institute for Social Medicine, Academic Medical Centre, Amsterdam

Introduction

'What are the common characteristics of interventions that are successful in reducing socioeconomic differences in health or in improving the health of the lowest socioeconomic groups?' Both the UK and the Netherlands have commissioned reviews of the literature to address this question.

The UK study, *Review of the Research on the Effectiveness of Health Services Interventions to Reduce Variations in Health,*[1] carried out by the NHS Centre for Reviews and Dissemination of York University in 1994, was commissioned by the Department of Health for its Variations in Health Sub-group of *The Health of the Nation* initiative. Its aim was to identify interventions which the NHS, either alone or in collaboration with other agencies, could use to improve the health of people from lower socioeconomic groups or ethnic minority groups or to reduce differences in health status. The review included only interventions with an experimental design (involving before and after studies with or without controls, randomised and non-randomised).

The Dutch review formed part of an overall programme carried out by the Programme Committee on Socioeconomic Health Inequalities in the Netherlands. The Programme, established in 1989, was set up to coordinate a research programme, investigate socioeconomic health differences and identify effective interventions that could form part of a strategy to address the problem. The Committee commissioned a literature review of interventions which have been shown to be effective. The aim was to identify common criteria for success that might inform the development of an intervention strategy. The literature search included interventions in various countries in Europe and North America, reported both in the traditional literature and the 'grey' literature.

There were two criteria for including intervention studies in the Dutch review: firstly that the intervention aimed to reduce ill health and in doing so reported outcome according to socioeconomic group; and secondly that the intervention had been evaluated. This second criterion posed problems as there were many different kinds of interventions and the quality of evaluation varied considerably.

An intervention was considered to have been effective in reducing social inequalities in coronary heart disease if it met at least one of two criteria: either that it had had a positive effect on health, or on a risk factor, that was at least as good in the lowest socioeconomic group as in other groups; or that the project had not widened the social class differential. Many of the 'easier' health education methods, such as mass media campaigns or simple written information, do not change behaviour in the 'hard to reach' groups. On the contrary, there is even evidence that these campaigns have increased the differences between socioeconomic groups.[2, 3]

This chapter concentrates on the conclusions that can be drawn from the Dutch review. It also looks at some of the similarities and differences between the two reviews, and examines the implications of the findings for policy and further research.

The range of interventions to reduce ill health

The UK and the Dutch reviews identified just under 100 interventions each, of which only 26 were common to both. Many of the interventions identified in the Dutch review did not meet the more rigorous criteria of the UK review. Also, many of the interventions identified in the UK review, but not included in the Dutch review, came from the United States. However, the characteristics of success were very similar in both reviews.

The Dutch review identified 98 interventions which aimed to reduce ill health and which reported outcomes according to socioeconomic group. These were analysed by the following criteria:
- target population
- intended effects of the intervention
- determinants of health which the intervention addressed
- the type of intervention method used
- the methods of evaluation, and
- the actual effects.

Some interventions were aimed at the general population; others were aimed at a specific population group such as children or women. Some were aimed at a specific disease or at particular risk factors. For example, 15 intervention programmes focused on coronary heart disease, or on the well known risk factors for coronary heart disease such as hypertension, diet, smoking cessation or physical activity. Other interventions were aimed at the more general determinants of health such as access to health care.

Effectiveness was rarely reported in terms of health outcome, but more frequently in terms of: a change in intermediary factors such as risk reduction or reduction in the prevalence of a risk factor; or an increase in the use of preventive or curative services; or a change in attitudes, knowledge or beliefs.

An intervention was deemed to be effective when the outcome measure showed a positive result and when it was at least as effective for the lowest socioeconomic groups as for the highest. Because the outcome measures and the socioeconomic status classifications differed between studies, it was very difficult to compare effectiveness. Costs of interventions were rarely measured.

Intervention methods used

The most commonly used intervention methods reported in the traditional scientific literature involved health education/promotion programmes, improving existing medical services, and making structural interventions (interventions which addressed factors beyond individual lifestyle, such as access to facilities, or policy change).

Small-scale local experiments

Most interventions identified in the Dutch review were small-scale. They included 31 intervention studies reported in the 'grey' literature, including local Healthy City projects, local health clinics, and groups working with specific communities. Many of these interventions were innovative. For example, in one study, lottery tickets were awarded to participants once they had achieved a certain improvement in the outcome being measured. This was a cheap and effective method of increasing uptake. The lottery ticket was cheap, per person, but the potential long-term population benefits were substantial.

While it is possible to learn lessons from these small-scale projects, they do not deliver a blueprint for a broad, effective intervention programme. Furthermore, many of these projects collapsed when funding ran out or when motivated individuals left the project. These studies showed that it is possible to reduce the inequalities in exposure to factors detrimental to health, but that this requires considerable long-term effort.

Determinants of health addressed by the interventions

Very few of the interventions identified in the literature review addressed the major determinants of health inequalities found in populations. The majority focused on lifestyle factors, or on effective use of existing medical services such as screening. Very few focused on the environmental or occupational determinants of health, although this may be partly because the search was conducted mainly within the medical and health literature. Some studies reported on structural measures such as reducing childhood accidents by setting up window guards. While such programmes may be extremely effective, they will not address the major causes of social inequalities in morbidity and mortality.

Evaluation of interventions

An additional problem arises with the evaluation of interventions, when their potential effects take a long time to manifest. Long time lags with, for instance, occupational exposure, may require sufficiently long follow-up periods, especially if different socioeconomic groups respond to the intervention at different rates.

Recording results by socioeconomic status

Very few of the projects were aimed specifically at reducing health inequalities. While some interventions were effective in reaching lower socioeconomic groups, they did not necessarily affect the gradient of health inequality.

Twenty of the 98 studies were aimed at all socioeconomic groups. Of these, 16 were at least as effective in the lower socioeconomic group as the highest. Sixty-eight studies were aimed specifically at lower socioeconomic groups. Of these, 35 were found to be effective.

It is recommended that, in future, research funding bodies should stipulate that outcome measures be reported not only by gender but also by socioeconomic status.

Characteristics of the most successful interventions

The most successful interventions identified in the Dutch review were:

- those that involved structural measures

- health education interventions that provided a combination of information and personal support, and

- interventions that provided a combination of health promotion and structural measures (see Table 1).

Table 1   *Types of intervention and their effectiveness*

Type of intervention	Effective	Dubious	Ineffective	Total
Structural measures	11 (69%)	4	1	16
Existing health care	5 (45%)	3	3	11
Health education and promotion:				
Providing information	6 (37%)	6	4	16
Providing information and personal support	32 (65%)	12	5	49
Health education and promotion and structural measures	2 (66%)	1	–	3
Other	2 (66%)	1	–	3
Total	58 (59%)	27	13	98

Source: See references 4 and 5.

Projects which are integrated with work already underway in the community are more likely to reach the target group than those which are not linked with existing services. Programmes that used existing health care services were more effective than one-off programmes. Local experiments are often driven by very committed individuals who move away once the funding comes to an end. If a project is to have a sustained effect in the long term, it may be necessary to 'institutionalise' it, that is incorporate it within an existing structure.

Large-scale intervention (or prevention) trials were usually as effective for lower as for higher socioeconomic groups: this may be because they are intensive programmes as opposed to the more general health education messages that are promoted in many of the traditional preventive programmes.

Among lower socioeconomic groups, the personal approach is more effective than simply providing written information. A general offer of information but without personal support leads to a greater uptake in the higher socioeconomic groups.

Conclusion

There is, as this review has shown, a paucity of intervention studies with well designed evaluation. Nevertheless, this should not deter the application of existing knowledge to policies which aim to reduce or at least prevent a further increase in socioeconomic differentials in health. Many of the interventions are small-scale, often started at local level in response to local need. This is excellent in terms of participatory health policy, but does not allow experience learnt from interventions to be systematically transferred to other settings. Funds should be allocated to well designed effectiveness studies, preferably randomised controlled trials, and preferably those which can be generalised to other risk factors and settings.

The interventions that are most successful in reducing the social inequalities in health are: interventions that involve structural measures; health education and promotion interventions that provide a combination of information and personal support; and interventions that provide a combination of health promotion and structural measures.

To enable the uptake of health promotion measures equally by all socioeconomic groups, it may be necessary to allocate resources unequally, targeting those most in need. Among lower socioeconomic groups, the personal approach is a much more effective method than simply providing written information. Reaching 'hard to reach' groups requires considerable extra investment in both time and money.

Intervention programmes must be integrated with existing health and social services if they are to be lasting and successful in the long term.

All research studies and NHS quality assurance programmes should examine the effect they have on different socioeconomic groups, in order to find out whether the programme has a greater impact on the most vulnerable. Grant-giving bodies should stipulate that studies should look at effectiveness in terms of socioeconomic status.

References

1 Arblaster L, Entwistle V, Lambert M, Foster M, Sheldon T, Watt I. 1995. *Review of the Research on the Effectiveness of Health Services Interventions to Reduce Variations in Health. CRD Report No. 3.* York: NHS Centre for Reviews and Dissemination.

2 Jackson C, Winkleby MA, Flora JA, Fortmann SP. 1991. Use of educational resources for cardiovascular risk reduction in the Stanford Five-City Project. *American Journal of Preventive Medicine*; 7: 82–8.

3 Wilkinson GS, Wilson J. 1983. An evaluation of demographic differences in the utilisation of cancer information service. *Social Science and Medicine*; 17: 169–175.

4 Gepkens A, Gunning-Shepers LJ. 1996. Interventions to reduce socioeconomic health differences. A review of the international literature. *European Journal of Public Health*; 6 (3): 218–226.

5 Gunning-Schepers LJ, Gepkens A. 1996. Reviews of interventions to reduce social inequalities in health: research and policy implications. *Health Education Journal*; 55: 226–238.

Acknowledgements

This chapter is by Professor Dr Louise Gunning-Schepers of the Institute for Social Medicine, Academic Medical Centre, Amsterdam, with additional material from 'Reviews of interventions to reduce social inequalities in health: research and policy implications', *a paper by Dr Gunning-Schepers and Annemiek Gepkens. For fuller details, see reference 5.*

Chapter 7

Smoking: patterns and policy options

Dr Alan Marsh

Policy Studies Institute

Introduction

The policy of increasing tobacco tax beyond the rate of inflation has helped to contribute to a reduction in the consumption of tobacco. However, the effect on the poorest smokers has been to increase hardship for them and their children.

The issues around tobacco tax and low income groups pose a familiar dilemma in health policy. There would be a valid cause for concern even if there were only small differences in the prevalence of smoking between the poor and the better off. In fact rates differ significantly: while smoking has halved among the better off families in Britain since the first General Household Survey in 1972,[1, 2] those on low incomes continue to smoke at the same high rates as in the 1970s.[3] This has opened up a large gap in prevalence between Britain's better off families compared with the poor.

Smoking is becoming concentrated among the poorest families, particularly among those with children. Twenty-seven per cent of smokers are concentrated in the lowest 10% income group. As a result, smoking prevalence is two to three times higher among the poorest groups compared even with those with middle-range incomes. Whereas average prevalence is down to just over a quarter in the UK, more than half those receiving income-tested benefits still regularly smoke cigarettes.

Other trends have coincided to aggravate the problem, for example:

- Several factors have increased the scale of poverty, notably the three-fold increase in lone parenthood from 500,000 to 1.7 million during the last 25 years and a doubling of long-term unemployment.[4] This has increased the absolute numbers of poor families in Britain. Also, these families have become relatively poorer compared to other families. Those in the lowest fifth of the income distribution have seen falls in real net disposable incomes after housing costs, while the real incomes of the top fifth have increased by 50%. There has been a strong polarisation in the standards of living of British families into one-fifth who have no earner at all and one-third who have two. During a time when the average family became nearly one-third better off, the proportion of British children in poverty increased from somewhere between 5% and 10% in 1979 (the variation depends on the measure used), to more than one in three in 1998. (See reference 5 for a detailed summary of the growth of income inequality in Britain.)

■ Tobacco control policy has increasingly relied on raising prices at twice the rate of inflation during a time when benefit incomes have been pegged to retail price inflation only. In 1997, the Chancellor of the Exchequer increased this rate to 5% over inflation, which had been typically running at 3%.

Variations in smoking rates

Social class differences

Using data from the General Household Survey, there *appears* to be a typical 'class diffusion model', with wealthier professionals being the first to accept the need to stop smoking following the Royal College of Physicians' report in 1962.[6] Subsequently, between 1972 and the early 1990s, smoking rates declined among all social groups (see Figure 1). However, among the higher occupational groups, the decrease started from a lower base: 32% of men in this group were smokers in 1972 compared to 65% of men in unskilled manual groups. Higher occupational groups have also maintained higher rates of smoking cessation than other occupational groups, and have much higher proportions of ex-smokers compared to ever-smokers.

Figure 1 *Cigarette smoking prevalence by sex and socioeconomic group, 1972–1990*

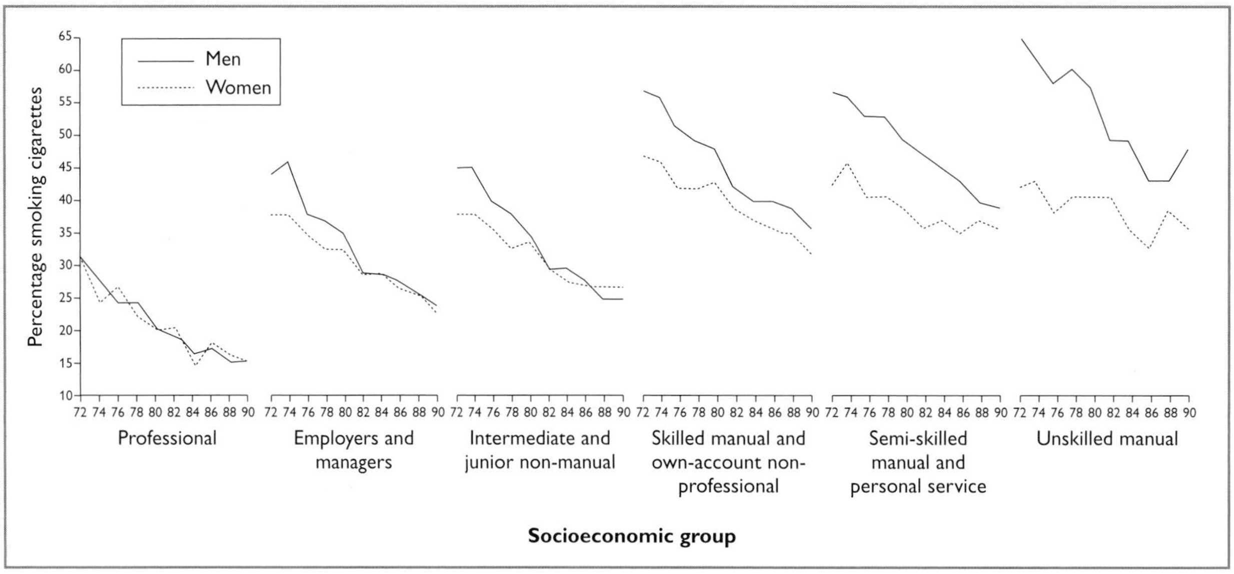

Source: See reference 7.

However, a fall in the percentage of smokers in some groups can be partly caused by differential mortality rates, which can cause an apparent fall in the numbers of smokers, particularly among unskilled manual men. If smokers continue to die of smoking-related diseases in large numbers while non-smokers survive longer and longer from the impact of improved post-war nutrition and health care, then the ratio of non-smokers to smokers will grow without anyone necessarily giving up smoking. There are two ways to become an ex-smoker.

It is therefore useful to examine the same prevalence rates for 16–44 year olds, as this eliminates the effect of differential mortality. It is also necessary to control for income rather than for social class which, for the majority of women, is recorded as for their husband's or partner's occupation. This analysis produces some striking results.

The basic pattern remains the same. The prevalence of smoking is declining among both men and women aged 16–44 in the highest income quarter and the second and third quarters. (see Figure 2). However, among those in the lowest income quarter there has been no change in prevalence: the proportion of smokers has remained at 50% since 1976. The proportion of lone parents who smoke has remained at 60% over the same period. The only change is that in 1990 there were three times as many lone parents as there were in 1976. There were also more poor couples with children.

Figure 2   *Changes in smoking prevalence, by income quarter and family type, among respondents aged 16–44, 1976–1990*

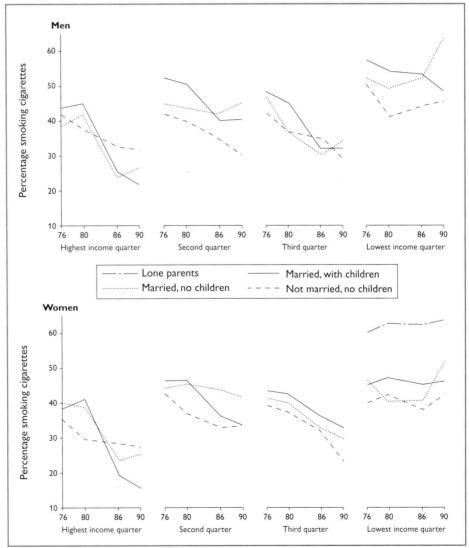

Source: See reference 3.

Variations between men and women

Smoking rates now differ very little between men and women. However, 73% of adults in low income families are women. High rates of smoking in this group are not associated with drinking: these women drink between one and two units of alcohol a week.[3]

Variations within low income groups

Not only is smoking concentrated among low income groups, but it is further concentrated among the most disadvantaged low income families. This pattern has hitherto remained invisible to official statistics.

For each marker of social disadvantage – social tenancy (living in council or housing association accommodation), having no educational qualifications and being in the habit of doing manual work – smoking levels almost double (see Table 1). The combined effects of these markers for disadvantage are very considerable. For example, among lone parents who are social tenants who have no qualifications and who do manual work, 69% are smokers, compared to just

Table 1 *Prevalence of smoking among lone parents, by tenancy, educational qualifications and type of work, 1991*

| | Percentages of lone parents who smoke | | | |
| | Owner-occupiers | | Social tenants | |
	Qualifications	No qualifications	Qualifications	No qualifications
Non-manual	29%	49%	37%	72%
Manual	44%	66%	71%	69%
No recent work	42%	30%	50%	61%

Source: See reference 3.

Table 2 *Prevalence of smoking among couples, by tenancy, educational qualifications and benefit status, 1991*

| | Percentages of people who smoke | | | |
| | Owner-occupiers | | Social tenants | |
	Qualifications	No qualifications	Qualifications	No qualifications
Women				
On IS or FC	28%	29%	48%	55%
Not on IS or FC	22%	30%	35%	49%
Men				
On IS or FC	36%	35%	53%	69%
Not on IS or FC	33%	37%	45%	51%
Both				
On IS or FC	21%	15%	33%	43%
Not on IS or FC	14%	16%	23%	29%

IS = Income Support   FC = Family Credit

Source: See reference 3.

over one-third of lone parents who are social tenants with qualifications and who do non-manual work. A lone parent living on means-tested benefits in council accommodation and who has no educational qualifications has an 84% chance of being a smoker, compared to 27% for young women nationally. Even among employed lone parents, such differences remain. Eleven per cent of lone parents who have paid jobs work as cleaners; 82% of them smoke.

Among couples, being on Income Support or Family Credit is a better indicator of smoking prevalence than qualifications (see Table 2). On the other hand, those who have become low-cost owner-occupiers with the same level of qualifications and type of work are no more likely to smoke than anyone else, and are significantly less likely to smoke than social tenants despite having similarly low income levels (at least at the time of asking). Council tenants who have been receiving means-tested benefits and who have no qualifications are between two and three times more likely to smoke than owner-occupiers in the same circumstances.

A problem of social geography

The important causal factor in continuing to smoke seems to be a persistently low trend income, or long-term poverty that is associated with a 'benefit fault line'. This is a new basis for multiple disadvantage in British society that is characterised by a combination of receipt of means-tested benefits (both in and out of work) and reliance on social housing. One hypothesis is that unqualified school leavers in the 1970s have been concentrated in council estates, which in turn have become isolated from the social trends which have influenced smoking behaviour in the mainstream of British society. Many of these school leavers have become Britain's low income families. Follow-up of the 1958 cohort in the National Child Development Study (NCDS)[3] found that nearly 60% of council tenants smoke compared to 24% of owner-occupiers (see Table 3).

Table 3 *Smoking rates by housing tenure and type of vendor (1958 cohort)*

Percentages of people who smoke

Tenure	Own outright	Buying on mortgage	Private tenant	Council tenant
	24%	27%	42%	59%
All owners Bought from:	Developer	Private	Housing association	Council
	18%	25%	34%	44%

Source: See reference 3.

Among those owner-occupiers who bought new homes from a developer, only 18% smoke (see Table 3) while among those who bought their homes under the 'right-to-buy' arrangements from the council, levels of smoking remain closer to those seen among continuing tenants (44% and 59% respectively). The effects of the differing social surroundings that characterise even the lower cost private housing compared with council estates seem to be a powerful constraint on smoking.

Social disadvantage as a barrier to quitting

Smoking is acquiring a new social profile. It follows the contours of disadvantage so closely [8, 9] that it is almost possible to study social disadvantage itself (even within low income groups) through variations in smoking practice. Does this mean that fewer young people from better off families, compared to those from poorer families, are taking up smoking nowadays, or that they are more likely to give up smoking as they get older?

The evidence from the NCDS data[3] suggests that both trends may be occurring but there is an interaction between people's family of origin and their own subsequent fortunes up to the age of 33 (the age at which the NCDS cohort was last interviewed in 1991). The percentage of young people taking up smoking is fairly similar across all social groups, though fewer among the best off homes start smoking. The difference is that those in higher income groups have a higher rate of giving up smoking, particularly among those who have children. Half the better off young smokers had given up by the age of 33 while only a quarter of the poorest fifth had managed to give up. This leaves prevalence among the poorest at twice that of the better off (see Table 4). Young smokers in the lowest income groups have a much lower rate of giving up smoking, especially if they subsequently have the experience of claiming Income Support. This is true even when lone parents are excluded from the analysis.

Table 4 *Smoking in the 1958 cohort: present income by past experience of income support, among two-parent families and those without children*

| | Percentage who smoke | | | | |
| | *Income quintile* | | | | |
	Lowest	2nd	3rd	4th	Highest
Two-parent families					
Claimed IS in the past					
Percentage who smoke	52%	44%	36%	36%	26%
Ex-smokers as a percentage of ever-smokers	25%	29%	39%	39%	48%
Never claimed IS					
Percentage who smoke	31%	30%	25%	21%	21%
Ex-smokers as a percentage of ever-smokers	38%	41%	48%	49%	52%
Cohort members without children					
Claimed IS in the past					
Percentage who smoke	50%	45%	39%	41%	26%
Ex-smokers as a percentage of ever-smokers	23%	20%	26%	24%	45%
Never claimed IS					
Percentage who smoke	45%	35%	34%	28%	26%
Ex-smokers as a percentage of ever-smokers	13%	31%	33%	40%	41%

IS = Income Support

Source: See reference 3.

This suggests that there is some binding factor which makes people cleave to smoking and to resist the trend to giving up in their 20s that clearly characterises other young people in the cohort. Poverty seems to be the key. Research on smoking cessation shows that success is associated with optimism.[10] The lack of an enduring means of family provision that they can control, the stress associated with this lack, the resulting feelings of inequality and indeed the fact of inequality, and the lack of opportunity, do not breed optimism. It is the sheer disappointment associated with missing out on the increases in living standards enjoyed by the majority that seems to bind young poor smokers to their habit and form a barrier to their giving up smoking.

The impact of smoking on the income of poor families

More than half of those on Income Support smoke and they spend about one-sixth of their net disposable income on cigarettes. After controlling for all other related factors, smoking is an additional cause of hardship for low income families. Couples who smoke are four and a half times more likely to be in severe hardship than other low income couples who do not smoke. Spending on cigarettes accounts for about one-third of this difference. The children of poor two-parent families where both the adults smoke are three times more likely to be going without essential items than the children of similarly poor families where the adults do not smoke.

From the 1991 figures, 16% of Income Support paid by the Department of Social Security for the support of adults who smoke is returned to the Treasury in the form of tobacco tax.[3] This amounted in 1991 to over £500 million in revenue paid by the most vulnerable group in society: poor families with children. Since 1991, this figure will have increased substantially as the real price of cigarettes has increased at twice the corresponding rate of increase in the purchasing power of social security benefits.

Tobacco control policy

The research poses a policy dilemma. Raising tobacco tax at twice to three times the rate of inflation is likely to reduce cigarette consumption among the majority. This is a good and entirely supportable policy. However, if the additional aim of tobacco tax policy is to reduce smoking among those who can least afford to smoke and among those of the poor who are anyway at greatest risk of smoking-related ill health, then new or additional policies are required.

While it is necessary to keep the price of cigarettes up to deterrent levels, a more clearly targeted policy to help low income smokers give up is needed. Tobacco control policies could be linked more securely to family welfare policy. Anti-smoking aids such as patches and gum could be available on prescription, making the means to give up smoking free for those who most need it. Targeting could be improved further by making such nicotine replacement therapies available as 'passported' benefits for those on means-tested social security benefits alongside other benefits such as free school meals, help with dental and optical testing costs. Community-based, outreach health promotion programmes are needed to back up such initiatives.

Tax is not levied on children's clothes or essential foodstuffs because it is argued that the poor should not have to pay tax. In fact the poor pay enormous sums of tax through tobacco tax. Some of the tobacco tax revenue paid by poor smokers on benefit could be mobilised to fund new, more appropriate ways of helping low income families give up smoking on a scale not previously attempted.

The future of smoking

If Britain is to meet its declared aim of reducing the prevalence of smoking to 20% by the year 2000, it is clear who the target group for action should be. For Britain's poor families, smoking is the norm. Only here are people still expected to smoke. The smaller numbers among them with more cause for optimism – the better qualified non-manual workers buying their homes – have already followed the national trend away from smoking.

If sufficient of the huge tax yield that poor smokers themselves contribute can be mobilised into a new assault on the problem, then an important opportunity arises. The resources could be ploughed back into a serious multi-level effort to break the hold that smoking has in poor communities, on a previously untried scale. The solution is not simply a question of increasing benefits or cash income: this would not address the community-based nature of the problem. The essential element will be to restore to Britain's poor and increasingly excluded families better reasons for optimism and some credible means to control their own lives. Welfare-to-work must be linked in turn to Welfare-to-health. Poor health is known to be a substantial barrier to work for many poor families – especially about 1 in 10 of lone parents.[11] Smoking itself is a barrier to work since so many workplaces now forbid their employees from smoking. Once people have a future they can believe in, one they value and therefore want to protect, giving up smoking becomes a credible and desirable goal.

If such a programme of change succeeds, then the national problem of smoking will be well on its way to resolution. Once smokers are a clear minority among this last host community for the habit, the trend will do the rest, just as it is doing among the better off. Once smoking has gone, it will not come back. One of the worst pandemics in the history of our national health will be over.

Conclusion

Cigarette smoking has become increasingly concentrated among low income groups. Smoking among middle and higher income groups has fallen during the past 25 years but has remained unchanged among the lowest income groups. Those living in social accommodation, claiming means-tested benefits, who are without educational qualifications and working in manual jobs, have rates of smoking twice to three times the national average of about one quarter. Social disadvantage, and the stress of inequality and social exclusion that now accompanies poverty, are major barriers to giving up smoking. The cost of smoking increases poor smokers' hardship and returns large amounts of social security benefit to the Treasury, posing a dilemma for tax policy.

Welfare-to-work measures should be accompanied by Welfare-to-health programmes that restore optimism to the lives of socially excluded poor groups, especially those with children such as lone parents.

References

1   *General Household Survey 1972.* 1973. London: HMSO.

2   See also: Wald N *et al.* 1988. *UK Smoking Statistics.* Oxford: Oxford University Press.

3   Marsh A, McKay S. 1994. *Poor Smokers.* London: Policy Studies Institute.

4   Haskey J. One parent families and their dependent children in Great Britain. In: Ford R, Millar J. 1998. *Private Lives and Public Responses: The Future of Lone Parent Policy in Britain.* London: Policy Studies Institute.

5   Goodman A, Johnson P, Webb S. 1997. *Inequality in the UK.* Oxford: Oxford University Press.

6   Royal College of Physicians. 1962. *Smoking and Health.* London: Pitman Medical.

7   Office of Population Censuses and Surveys. 1991. *General Household Survey: Cigarette Smoking 1972 to 1990,* OPCS Smoking Monitor, 26. November, ss 91/3.

8   Graham H. 1988. Women and smoking in the United Kingdom: the implications for health promotion. *Health Promotion;* 4: 371–382.

9   Graham H. 1992. *Smoking Among Working Class Mothers with Children.* Unpublished, Department of Health.

10 Marsh A, Matheson J. 1983. *Smoking Attitudes and Behaviour.* London: HMSO.

11 Ford R, Marsh A, Finlayson L. 1997. *Lone Parents, Work and Benefits. Research Report No. 61.* London: The Stationery Office.

12 Office of Population Censuses and Surveys. 1991. *Family Spending in 1991.* London: HMSO.

13 Office of Population Censuses and Surveys. 1978. *Family Expenditure Survey, 1976.* London: HMSO.

Acknowledgements

This chapter is based on Poor Smokers,[3] *a report on the impact of smoking on the welfare of low income families and their children. Jointly funded by the Health Education Authority and the Department of Social Security, the report draws on four sources: new analysis of the Department of Social Security/Policy Studies Institute survey of 2,200 low income families (including further follow-up of a cohort of 900 lone parents and 500 very low income families); new analysis of the OPCS General Household Surveys for 1976, 1980, 1986 and 1990; OPCS Family Expenditure Surveys over the same period;[12, 13] and the National Child Development Study.*

Chapter 8

Nutrition: patterns and policy options

Ms Suzi Leather

Food policy consultant

Introduction

Coronary heart disease seriously affects life expectancy and health, but it does not affect all people equally. There are marked differences in the incidence of coronary heart disease between different socioeconomic groups. One of the reasons for this variation is the difference in behavioural risk factors, one of which is nutrition.

There are many dietary factors that have been linked to risk of coronary heart disease, which may help explain the relatively higher risks of the disease among lower socioeconomic groups.

The links between a diet rich in saturated fat are well recognised: saturated fat raises serum cholesterol, a known risk factor for coronary heart disease; trans-fatty acids from hydrogenated margarines contribute to thrombosis and atherogenesis, together with a low intake of long-chain polyunsaturated n-3 fatty acids which come from oily fish.

More recently, low intakes of antioxidants, such as beta-carotene and vitamin C, which are found in fruit and vegetables, have been linked to atherogenesis. Also homocysteinuria, induced by folate intakes below 400 micrograms a day, has been shown as an independent risk factor for coronary heart disease, stroke and peripheral vascular disease.

There are marked variations between socioeconomic groups in Britain in some of the dietary factors associated with coronary heart disease and these dietary variations mirror variations in the incidence of the disease. For example Scotland, which has among the highest premature mortality rates from coronary heart disease in the world, has one of the lowest vegetable and fruit intakes. Moreover, regional variations in fruit and vegetable intake within Scotland relate to regional differences in coronary heart disease.[1]

Overall the UK population gets less of its energy from fruit and vegetables than almost any other Western European country (see Figure 1).

Figure I *Fruit and vegetable consumption in Europe, 1992*

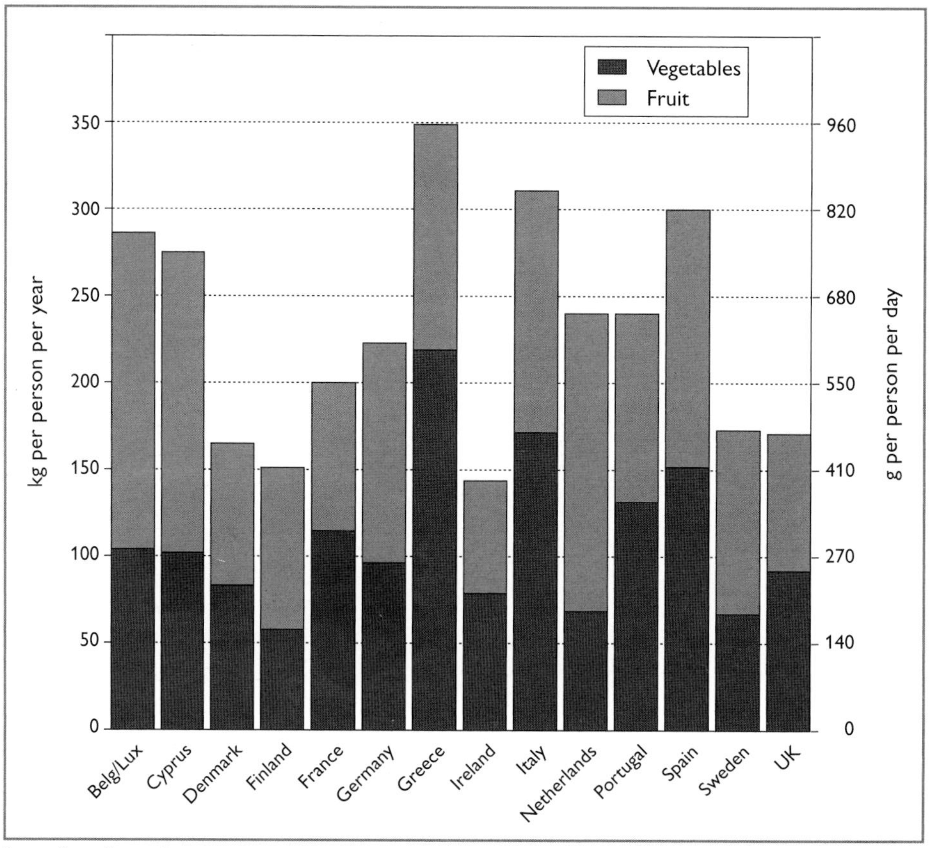

Source: See reference 2.

Socioeconomic differences in food and nutrition intake

The annual National Food Survey[3] of 8,000 British households shows that, compared with the highest income group (A), households in the lowest income group (D and E2*) consume more milk (but less semi-skimmed milk), meat and meat products (of which more is higher fat meat products), fats, sugars and preserves, potatoes and cereals. They also consume fewer fresh vegetables, fruit and higher fibre products such as brown and wholewheat bread, ie foods which have a higher nutrient density.

Comparing intake of nutrients as a percentage of the reference nutrient intake** across different income groups, the evidence shows that intake of most nutrients that protect against coronary heart disease is lower in socioeconomic groups D and E2, and markedly so for calcium, iron, magnesium, folate and especially vitamin C. Also, intake of fibre is much lower.[4] (See Figures 2 and 3.)

There is little variation by socioeconomic group in the percentage intake of food energy derived from fat, but there are differences in the ratio of polyunsaturated to unsaturated fats (the P:S ratio) with lower socioeconomic groups having a lower P:S ratio.[4]

---

*   In 1995 income group A was defined as households with a gross weekly income of more than £570. Income group D/E2 was defined as households with a gross weekly income of less than £140.

**   The level that prevents 97.5% of the population from developing a classic deficiency.

Figure 2 *Variation in vitamin C intake by socioeconomic group*

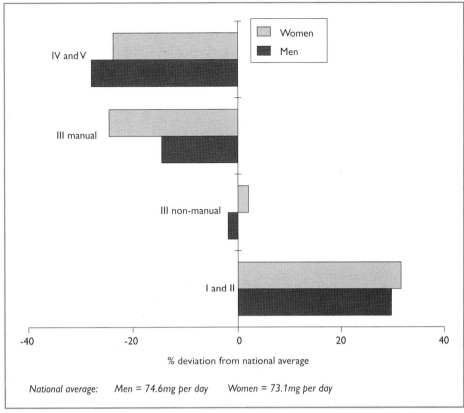

Source: See reference 4.

Figure 3 *Variation in carotene intake by socioeconomic group*

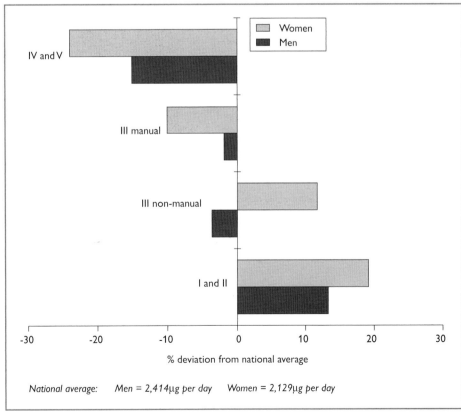

Source: See reference 4.

Impact of household size

The already low UK average consumption of fruit and vegetables hides a marked variation between the different income groups. These nutritional inequalities are further intensified when the effects of family size are also considered (see Table 1).

Table I   *The impact of income and family size on consumption of some foods relevant to the development of coronary heart disease*

| | Families with I child | | Families with 4 or more children | |
| | Income band | | Income band | |
Foods (grams per person per week)	A	D/E2	A	D/E2
Potatoes	523	744	353	860
Fresh green vegetables	255	143	143	98
Other fresh vegetables	683	289	420	350
Processed vegetables	455	644	345	718
Fresh fruit	653	329	588	261
Other fruit/products	574	280	497	109
All fats	171	182	147	314
Sugar/preserves	127	190	317	204
Fish	139	88	88	68

Source: See reference 3.

The 1991 National Children's Home survey[5] found that, in a sample of families attending their family centres, one in five parents and one in ten children had gone without food in the previous month because of lack of money. It is not just about going without, but about keeping up and being unable to maintain the food expectations of the majority. The diets of people on a low income are typically characterised by their lack of variety. This is problematic since, in addition to compromising the diet particularly in terms of micronutrients, there is the added psychological stress of being excluded from the widely accepted and promoted expectations of society.

Taking vegetables as an example: excluding potatoes, low income households eat considerably less fresh vegetables than those of higher income.[6] Low income households buy the cheaper items – cabbage and root vegetables – rather than beans, peas, broccoli, and leafy salads. Even so, they still eat over one-fifth less fresh vegetables overall compared to rich households. The fresh green vegetable consumption of people in the poorest quarter of households in Britain is the equivalent, on average, of only three Brussels sprouts a day (only one-third of a portion). People from the largest poor families consume even less fresh green vegetables – on average, the equivalent of less than a couple of sprouts a day.

The variations in fruit consumption are even more marked. Overall, people in income band D/E2 consume one-third less fresh fruit than those in band A. Families in the poorest income group D/E2 consume, on average, the equivalent

Figure 4 *Fresh fruit consumption by family size and income, 1994*

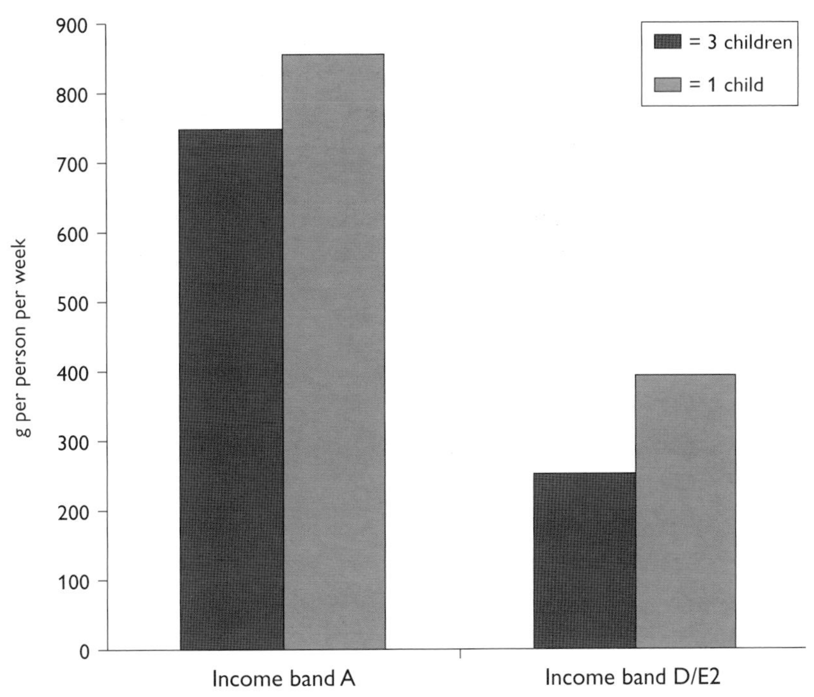

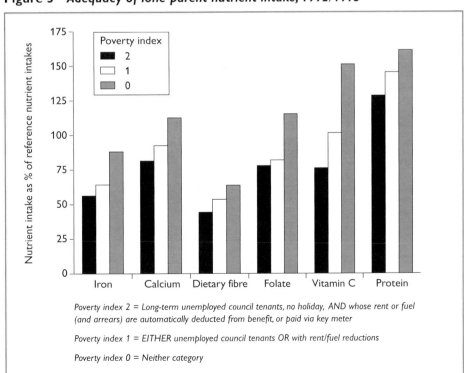

Source: See reference 7.

of less than half an orange a day. The gap between households in different socioeconomic groups is intensified once children are present. Families with children in income group A consume two to three times the amount of fresh fruit compared with families in income band D/E2. The total fresh fruit consumption of people in large poor families is the equivalent, on average, of only a quarter of an orange a day.

Figure 5 *Adequacy of lone parent nutrient intake, 1992/1993*

Poverty index 2 = Long-term unemployed council tenants, no holiday, AND whose rent or fuel (and arrears) are automatically deducted from benefit, or paid via key meter

Poverty index 1 = EITHER unemployed council tenants OR with rent/fuel reductions

Poverty index 0 = Neither category

See reference 8.

Socioeconomic differences in children's fruit consumption begin early in life. Within their first year, infants from ABC1 families eat 50% more fruit than their C2DE peers.[9] As the number of children in the higher income households rises, so the amount of fruit consumed per person rises. It is the reverse for low income families: fruit consumption declines with each additional child. The fresh fruit consumption of the largest low income families is the equivalent of only a quarter of an apple per person a day. Many children eat even less fruit, often not even every week. In Scotland, the proportion of children eating fresh fruit less than once a week ranges from 19% to 27%.[1]

Nutritional deprivation impacts more on women, partly because poverty impacts more on women, and partly because women bear the brunt of food poverty within families. Analysis of the government's *Dietary and Nutritional Survey of British Adults* found that more than one in four women in households receiving benefits had diets deficient in iron, vitamin A, thiamin, riboflavin, vitamin B6 and vitamin C.[4] The extent of this inadequacy has been illustrated in a nutritional study of lone parent families[8] (see Figure 5).

Trends

Over the past 15 years, food consumption and energy intakes have fallen, reflecting an increasingly sedentary lifestyle. This means that diets need to be more nutrient-dense to compensate. However, people from higher socioeconomic groups seem more able to compensate than people from lower socioeconomic groups and there is a growing gap between the nutrient density of the diet of the two groups.[10]

Some large families on a low income now eat, by weight, twice as much sugar as they do fresh green vegetables, and more fat than fresh fruit. In recent years the consumption of fresh green vegetables among lower socioeconomic groups has fallen considerably. In larger families on low income, the consumption of fresh green vegetables has fallen to one-third of its 1980 level.* The intake of antioxidants among the poorest of households has declined dramatically since 1980: intake of beta-carotene has fallen by 47% and vitamin C by 23%.[11]

The nutrition gap between socioeconomic groups is widening, and it is the foods with health-protective effects which show the greatest inequalities in consumption.

The scale of the problem

The UK has no official, or unofficial, food deprivation index, so it is difficult to put exact numbers on the scale of the problem of inadequate diet. However, it can be said with absolute confidence that the numbers at risk of nutritional ill health have risen dramatically since the end of the 1970s because of the greater numbers of people living in poverty.

---

*   For a more detailed analysis of trends see 'What changes in national policy could improve children's eating patterns?' by S. Leather in *Food for Children*, published by the National Heart Forum, 1994.

Without entering into the thorny debate about the meaning and extent of poverty, it is possible to make some calculations of the scale of nutritional ill health by looking at income levels and considering the food expenditure patterns typical at, or below, these levels.

The National Food Survey shows the food spending patterns of the population divided by income with (in 1995), D and E2 being households with gross weekly incomes of under £140.[5] Average daily per capita consumption of fresh fruit and vegetables in these households is the equivalent of less than half an orange and only one-third of a portion of vegetables. In 1995, 24% of UK households were living on incomes below £140 per week. Therefore, it can reasonably be argued that this level of consumption of fruit and vegetables is typical for almost a quarter of the population; they are not even eating one portion of fresh fruit and vegetables a day.

In terms of policy interventions, it is particularly important to note that the composition of households living with this level of dietary inadequacy has changed to comprise more young, single householders, fewer pensioner couples and single pensioners and many more couples with children.[12] There is evidence that parents' nutritional intakes are markedly inadequate when they face deductions from benefit (for example from fuel and water rates arrears), as one in five claimants do.[8]

The reasons for dietary inequalities

It is tempting for many to blame the poor themselves for choosing low quality, unhealthy diets but there are other explanations which have practical solutions.[13]

- Low income families have less access to large-scale retailers which, because of economies of scale, can provide a wider variety of affordable foods which make up a healthy diet compared with small local retailers.[14, 15]

- A varied and healthy diet, however defined, consistently costs more than a monotonous, unhealthy diet. Healthy eating is not cheaper than a typical poor diet.[16]

- Healthy food costs more in deprived areas than in richer ones and is often of inferior quality.[17]

- Those on a low income already spend a higher percentage of their income on food.

- Many cheap, high calorie foods are also high in fat and sugar.

- There are little or no significant differences between the levels of knowledge about healthy eating between different income groups.[18]

- Low income consumers are actually more efficient purchasers of nutrients than those with higher incomes.[19]

- There is no evidence that low income consumers are less skilled in preparing and cooking food than higher income consumers, although there is mounting concern that there is a considerable deficit in cooking skills across all socioeconomic groups. It is certainly the case that the poorer you are the more skill is required to manage a wholly inadequate income. The skills deficit therefore has a greater impact on those on low income.

These factors combine to promote the risk of coronary heart disease among lower socioeconomic groups. Recent evidence shows that type of neighbourhood is associated with risk factors such as poorer diet, smoking and physical activity, independently of social class, and household income. This suggests that more attention needs to be paid to characteristics of local neighbourhoods as well as individuals living within them.[15]

The real reason for dietary inequalities lies with that pernicious matrix: inadequate income and reduced entitlements to benefits such as free school meals, inadequate access and facilities, the deficit in cooking skills, and overwhelming commercial pressure for foods which promote an unhealthy diet. All must be addressed to make healthy eating the easy choice.

Recommendations

From the point of view of coronary heart disease and diet, the aim must be to improve the diets of the most disadvantaged, principally by increasing fruit and vegetable consumption, and altering the P:S ratio. But these aims are inseparable from the overall problems of inadequate income, access, and cooking skills, none of which will be addressed just with the provision of more advice and information.

International policy

- *The Common Agricultural Policy should be reformed.*

The Common Agricultural Policy (CAP) needs to be reformed, in particular the regime which currently inflates European Union prices of fruit and vegetables and penalises third country imports. The impact of the CAP on food prices has a disproportionately greater effect on people on a low income who are more dependent on foods covered by the CAP.[20]

European Union food and agricultural policy should place more emphasis on nutritional value, for example by promoting diversity and production of foods containing higher levels of antioxidants. There should be more emphasis placed on the consumption of fruit and vegetables with a reduction in excess dairy fat production. Support for European fruit and vegetable growers needs to be through direct income aid to growers, not through higher food prices.

National policy

- *Income should be maximised, to address poverty and deprivation.*

In October 1993, a review of the academic literature presented to the government's Nutrition Task Force concluded that there was a real food poverty problem to be addressed, and explicitly rejected the ignorance explanation, instead focusing on issues such as the inadequacy of state benefits.[16] Policies to tackle dietary inequalities will have to address the material basis of poverty and deprivation.

The Department of Social Security (DSS) does not disclose the contribution of the food component to benefit levels which, in any case, are not calculated on the basis of needs. However, there is indisputable evidence about the inadequacy of benefit levels. As nutritional needs vary, so should the value of the food element.

There is a particular need to give more to pregnant women on low incomes,[21] people who require special diets, and families living in bed and breakfast accommodation. In 1995, the cost of an adequate diet for a pregnant woman was calculated as nearly 40% of the total income of a single woman over 25 years on benefit, nearly 50% of the benefit of an 18–24 year old woman, and nearly 65% for a pregnant woman aged 16–17 years (although they are eligible for income support only during the last 11 weeks of pregnancy).[21] Other research has implicated poor maternal diet with the development of heart disease in later life.[22] Rarely can medical and social science have jointly presented such a compelling case for social policy reform.

There is another advantage to having an explicit food element in benefit levels. Debt is closely related to poor diet. Expenses such as fuel and water arrears, housing costs, local tax, child support orders and social fund loans may be deducted from benefit. There is effectively no upper limit on the amount that can be deducted, so there is a continual erosion of the amount left for the only flexible item in the budget – food. This explains why, in so many low income families, food expenditure is so low.[23]

Several European countries make an annual calculation of what families need to live on. This figure can then be used not only to set benefits, but by courts as a minimum level below which debt repayments cannot be enforced.

- *Local food projects should be encouraged, supported and financed.*

Local food projects such as co-ops represent both a sign of the problem (in that they are organised in areas of deprivation suffering from a lack of access), and a possible solution. Food co-ops are community-based, bulk-buy schemes which enable consumers to have access to good quality food, especially fruit and vegetables, at between one-third and a half of shop prices. They also provide psychosocial support. The National Food Alliance has collated examples of such initiatives.[24] But local projects cannot get finance from central government departments, and local authorities' budgets are being squeezed; likewise non-mandatory grants to voluntary bodies have been cut. There is an urgent need to secure funding for local projects – funding which is sustained and independent of commercial bias.

- *Low income women who choose to breastfeed should be given an extra dietary allowance.*

At present women on Income Support are entitled to free formula milk. This is an important benefit, but without some financial support for breastfeeding women, the financial incentive contradicts the health message.

- *Commercial pressures on children should be restricted.*

Many children live in families whose principal, or in some cases only, source of entertainment is television. Many children are exposed to advertisements for high fat, high sugar foods. The food industry must be required to accept a tougher code of advertising, particularly as regards children. In 1993 only £2.9 million was spent advertising fresh fruit and vegetables and nuts. Nearly 25 times more was spent on advertising chocolate. For the food industry, this is money well spent: while nearly half of school children eat two or more chocolate bars or sweets each day, one in four have no fresh fruit or vegetables at all.[25] Commercial pressures have a particular impact on the most nutritionally vulnerable, as children of parents who cannot afford other forms of entertainment spend more time watching television.

- *Social fund grants, rather than loans, should be provided for essential items such as a cooker or fridge.*

Community workers report that some children cannot play traditional mealtime games because they are unfamiliar with the notion of sitting down to a meal and may not even have a table and chair at home. For too many people, meals are what you eat between the chip shop and the front door. Sometimes the reason for this is simply lack of cooking facilities. Although most people would agree that a cooker or fridge are essential items, the DSS does not. At the moment even a cooker is not regarded as essential. Families may therefore be refused a loan to buy one.

- *VAT should not be imposed on food.*

VAT on food would be a regressive tax, because the poor spend a greater percentage of their income on food.

- *There should be subsidies rather than levies on healthy foods.*

New ways to increase consumption by making healthier foods cheaper should be developed. This was achieved successfully in Norway with fruit and vegetables, cereals and low fat milk.

Schools and education

- *Free school meals, including breakfast, at minimum nutritional standards should be supplied, as well as free fruit and milk at school.*

This would have overwhelming support from parents. If this is deemed to be too expensive then it could at least be targeted to schools in deprived areas.

- *Schools should give out consistent messages about healthy eating.*

The right overall environment has to be created for healthy eating: saying one thing in the classroom and then surrounding children with conflicting messages, particularly from commercial sponsors, is clearly inappropriate.

- *Cooking skills should be included in the national curriculum.*

This would give all children the opportunity to learn food preparation and cooking skills, meal planning and food budgeting. While it is up to parents to pass on skills to their children, they cannot pass on knowledge they do not have. There is a generation of people many of whom no longer know how to cook. Without the ability to cook, people are more dependent on convenience foods which are more expensive. Again the poor are harder hit.

- *Adults should be encouraged to acquire the skills and the confidence to cook.*

Some parents do not have the confidence to cook for their children because the children expect food to taste like tinned or packet food, and anything else seems 'wrong'. Some healthy eating initiatives have tried to give peer group support to bolster confidence in cooking skills, as well as offering information on cheap sources of important nutrients.

Health authorities

- *The emphasis on individual behavioural change should be augmented with social action.*

Dietary change needs social and psychological support. Health authorities should employ the principle of subsidiarity: health education is best done at the level closest to the local communities – ideally from places to which people already look for support, such as community and family centres and schools.

- *Health education agencies should recognise poor people's most immediate concern – lack of money.*

Poor people are more concerned about this week's debts than about the health consequences in 30 years' time.

Local authorities

- *Opportunities for supporting local food shops should be explored.*

Few of the poorest families have access to a private car, but retailers have been moving out of town and the total number of retail outlets has declined by 35% since 1980. Between 1986 and 1992, a quarter of greengrocers closed. Food at local shops is, on average, 23% more expensive than in supermarkets.[14]

These developments are drawing food retailing out of the cities to the periphery, leaving inner city areas and many housing estates facing substantial food retailing problems. Alternatively, the developers should be made to bear some of the costs they presently impose on people on low income. For example, planning permission could be made dependent on the retailers providing a free bus service from areas of poor housing, or developers could be required to provide equivalent shelf space in poorer areas.

Attention needs to be paid to measures and incentives which will enable local shops to function competitively in the food economy. These could include tax and rate rebates and, in many areas with high levels of crime, security arrangements for premises and shop personnel.

Local development and planning bodies need to encourage more street and local markets, as well as local shops selling good quality healthy food. Fruit and vegetable stalls are particularly needed. These could be encouraged by differential rating or leasing tariffs. These retail outlets should be targeted at deprived areas.

- *Local authorities should provide more free allotments.*

Under the 1950 Allotment Act, every local authority has an obligation to provide four acres of allotments per 1,000 population. This could go some way to enabling some low income families to eat more fruit and vegetables.[26]

Industry

- *Healthier foods should be included in the 'price war'.*

Healthier foods are not generally included in the price war, and foods which are unrefined often cost more than their refined equivalents. These price incentives must be reversed.[27]

- *Profit margins on foods in the UK should be reduced.*

Food prices are higher in the UK than in other European countries, and mark-ups by UK food retailers are comparatively high. Profit margins in the UK are as high as 8%, compared with about 2% in Europe and as low as 1% in the United States. Such profit levels cannot be justified in a country such as the UK which has one of the highest and fastest growing levels of poverty in Europe.

Conclusion

Socioeconomic differences in coronary heart disease can in part be accounted for by diet. The diet of lower socioeconomic groups provides cheap energy from foods such as meat products, full-fat milk, fats and sugar, and is relatively low in intake of fruit and vegetables, oily fish, and fibre-rich starchy products. This type of diet is lower in essential nutrients such as calcium, iron, magnesium, folate, vitamin C and beta-carotene than that of higher socioeconomic groups. In addition to the nutritional concerns, the cumulative effect of inadequate access and income creates great stress which, in turn, may be a contributing factor to coronary heart disease. There is scope for enormous health gain if the diet of lower socioeconomic groups could be changed through a variety of measures which would promote access to a healthier diet. Policies need to be tailored towards the needs of communities in addition to changing individual behaviour. The cost implications of ignoring these factors and the interrelationship between them is a high price in terms of human happiness, and an enormously inflated NHS bill.

References

1   The Scottish Office. 1993. *The Scottish Diet. Report of a Working Party to the Chief Medical Officer for Scotland*. Edinburgh: The Scottish Office Home and Health Department/HMSO Scotland.

2   Food and Agriculture Organization Agrostat Supply Data. Cited in: Williams C. Recommendations and current consumption patterns: how big is the gap? In: Sharp I (ed.) 1997. *At Least Five A Day: Strategies to Increase Vegetable and Fruit Consumption*. London: The Stationery Office.

3   Ministry of Agriculture, Fisheries and Food. 1996. *National Food Survey, 1995*. London: HMSO.

4   Ministry of Agriculture, Fisheries and Food. 1994. *The Dietary and Nutritional Survey of British Adults: Further Analysis*. London: HMSO.

5   National Children's Home. 1991. *Poverty and Nutrition Survey 1991*. London: National Children's Home.

6   All details on consumption by large poor families are taken from unpublished data from the *National Food Survey, 1992*. The author is grateful to the Ministry of Agriculture, Fisheries and Food for providing additional data.

7   Ministry of Agriculture, Fisheries and Food. 1995. National Food Survey 1994. London: HMSO.

8   Dowler E, Calvert C. 1995. *Nutrition and Diet in Lone-parent Families*. London: Family Policy Studies Centre.

9   Mills A, Tyler H. *Food and Nutrient Intakes of British Infants Aged 6–12 Months*. London: Ministry of Agriculture, Fisheries and Food/HMSO.

10 James WPT et al. 1997. The contribution of nutrition to inequalities in health. *British Medical Journal*; 314: 1545–1549.

11 Leather S, Dowler E. 1997. Intake of micronutrients in Britain's poorest fifth has declined. *British Medical Journal*; 314: 1412.

12 Oppenheim C, Harker L. 1996. *Poverty: The Facts*. London: Child Poverty Action Group.

13 Low Income Project Team, 1996. *Health of the Nation: Low Income, Food, Nutrition and Health: Strategies for Improvement. A Report of the Low Income Project Team for the Nutrition Task Force*. London: HMSO.

14 Pichaud D, Webb J. 1996. *The Price of Food: Missing Out on Mass Consumption*. London: STICERD.

15 Ellaway A, MacIntyre S.1996. Does where you live predict health related behaviours? A case study in Glasgow. *Health Bulletin*; 54 (6): 443–446.

16 Dowler E, Rushton C. 1994. *Diet and Poverty in the UK. Contemporary Research Methods and Current Experience: A Review. Publication no 11*. London: Department of Public Health and Policy, London School of Hygiene and Tropical Medicine, University of London.

17 Leather S. 1992. Less money, less choice: Poverty and diet in the UK today. In: National Consumer Council (ed). *Your Food: Whose Choice?* London: HMSO.

18 Health Education Authority. 1989. *Diet, Nutrition and 'Healthy Eating' in Low Income Groups*. London: Health Education Authority.

19 Cole-Hamilton I. 1988. *Review of Food Patterns Amongst Lower Income Groups in the UK*. Unpublished report to the Health Education Authority.

20 Leather S. 1997. *The CAP, diet and nutrition: A consumer view. In: The CAP, Diet and Nutrition*: Seminar organised by the Consumers in Europe Group, Department of Agriculture and Food Economics, University of Reading.

21 NCH Action for Children/Maternity Alliance. 1995. *Poor Expectations. Poverty and Undernourishment in Pregnancy*. London: NCH Action for Children/Maternity Alliance.

22 Barker DJP (ed). 1992. *Foetal and Infant Origins of Adult Diseases*. London: British Medical Journal Books.

23 National Consumer Council. 1995. *Budgeting for Food on Benefits*. London: National Consumer Council.

24 National Food Alliance. 1994. *Low Income Pack. A Practical Guide for Advisers and Supporters Working with Families and Young People on Low Incomes*. London: National Food Alliance.

25 Williams C, Ward P. 1993. *School Meals. Report of a Survey of Parents' Attitudes to the School Meals Service, and Weekday Dietary Habits of Children in Seven Case Study Schools*. London: Consumers' Association.

26 National Food Alliance. 1996. *Growing Food in Cities Project*. London: National Food Alliance.

27 Brockbank D, Lobstein T. 1995. Fruit and vegetables don't figure much in budget food in supermarket. *Food Magazine*; 28; 3: 11–13.

Ms Suzi Leather is an individual member of the National Heart Forum.

Chapter 9

Physical activity: patterns and policy options

Professor Ken Roberts

Department of Sociology, Social Policy and Social Work Studies, University of Liverpool

Adrian Field

Assistant Director, National Heart Forum

Introduction

Physical activity is one of the 'best buys' in public health, including coronary heart disease prevention. However, the social inequalities prevalent in other coronary heart disease risk factors such as smoking and nutrition (see Chapters 7 and 8) are also reflected in data on physical activity. Addressing inequalities in physical activity requires a cross-sectoral approach that targets deprived areas, especially children in low socioeconomic groups.

The benefits of physical activity

There is clear evidence that physical inactivity is an independent risk factor for coronary heart disease among men, and that regular physical activity can reduce this risk.[1] Men who are physically active have half the risk of coronary heart disease of those who are sedentary. The relative risk of coronary heart disease associated with low levels of activity is similar to the risk associated with classic risk factors such as smoking, high blood pressure and high blood cholesterol. Although insufficient research has been carried out among women to establish whether the same relationship holds for women, there is evidence that physical activity can modify some of the risk factors in women, such as high blood pressure, cholesterol levels and obesity.[2]

The benefits of physical activity are not restricted to vigorous activity, but are graded: more activity, in terms of time and intensity, confers a greater health benefit.[3] Thirty minutes' activity of moderate intensity on most days of the week can protect against coronary heart disease. Examples include brisk walking, cycling, dancing and swimming.[4]

About two-thirds of the population in the UK could benefit from increased levels of physical activity. At present, 64% of men and 76% of women are either sedentary or are moderately active on an irregular basis only.[5]

Physical activity protects not only against coronary heart disease but also against other chronic and disabling conditions, including overweight and obesity, stroke, hypertension, non-insulin dependent diabetes mellitus, osteoporosis and cancer of the colon.[3]

Inequalities in levels of physical activity

Inequalities in levels of physical activity are clearly evident in relation to education, housing tenure and employment indicators. However, an examination of the relationship between physical activity levels and social class produces mixed results.

Education

The National Fitness Survey found that greater numbers of people with educational or professional qualifications to GCE 'O' level standard or equivalent, particularly among the oldest age group, participated in activities of moderate or vigorous intensity, compared to those with lower or no qualifications.[5]

Housing tenure

Using housing tenure as a social indicator, 28% of men and 23% of women living in rented council accommodation have a sedentary lifestyle compared to 15% of male and 14% of female owner-occupiers, and 14% of men and 19% of women in privately rented homes.[5]

Employment status

There are striking differences in activity patterns between unemployed men and those in work (see Figure 1). Higher proportions of men designated 'unemployed and seeking work' are sedentary, and lower proportions are regularly active at a moderate intensity level or above, compared with those who are in work. The 'other' category includes people who are not in employment for health reasons, so the lower levels of activity are to be expected. The differentials for women are less clear.[6] In the UK, as in most Western countries since the 1960s, two sections of the population where participation in sport is particularly low are retired people and the unemployed.[7] Being out of employment clearly does not necessarily equate with undertaking even moderate levels of physical activity.

Social class

However, in terms of social class differentials in physical activity levels, the picture is mixed.[5, 6] Slightly higher proportions of social class V men and women are sedentary compared with those in other classes, and half as many are active on a regular vigorous basis. However, higher proportions of men in manual classes are active on a regular, moderate basis. Data for women show less variation between the social classes.[6]

On the other hand, some surveys do show a social class gradient in leisure time physical activity. Lower rates of physical activity were found in manual compared to non-manual groups in both the South and the North of Great Britain in 1985 and 1992 (see Figure 2). Furthermore, although the percentage of men and women taking part in physical activity increased over that period, the social differentials remained.

The explanation for the mixed survey findings is that there are higher participation rates in higher social classes for leisure time activities, but this is largely balanced out by higher physical activity levels in manual classes during work time, which takes place on most of the week.

Figure 1 *Participation at different activity levels by employment status, men aged 16–64, England, 1990–1991*

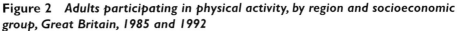

'Other' includes people who are not in employment for health reasons.

Source: See reference 6.

Figure 2 *Adults participating in physical activity, by region and socioeconomic group, Great Britain, 1985 and 1992*

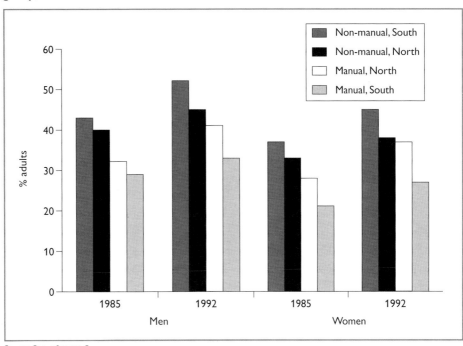

Source: See reference 8.

Ethnicity

There are also lower levels of involvement in sports-based activities among those of Afro-Caribbean, Indian, Pakistani and Bangladeshi origin than among the UK population as a whole.[9]

Children

School children are mostly insufficiently active for the good of their health,[10, 11] and the patterns of inequality in levels of physical activity are also apparent among children. A survey by the Health Education Authority found that children from lower socioeconomic groups did less exercise on average that other children. Working class families are less likely to introduce their children to leisure time physical activity. Children from lower socioeconomic classes reported less exercise outside school than those from higher socioeconomic classes.[12] By adulthood, the patterns of physical activity are well established and thereafter are unlikely to change.

However, there is little evidence of social class inequalities among school children in terms of taking part in *sports*. Participation in sport by school pupils does not appear to be the domain of any specific social group. Also, it appears that, despite exhortations to concentrate on traditional team sports, the broad sports curricula in schools encourages greater participation in sports through access to a wide range of sports during school education.[13] The increase in the numbers of young people in post-compulsory education has also contributed to an increase in participation in sport among young people.

Participation in sports

Despite these inequalities in physical activity, people in all sociodemographic groups are more likely to be 'sports active' today than their counterparts of 20 and 30 years ago.[14] Involvement in sport is, however, only one aspect of physical activity. The divergence in *overall* levels of physical activity is a cause for concern, particularly in view of the wider use of cars and labour-saving devices.

Moreover, participation in sport is unlikely to eliminate or even reduce social class health inequalities. Sport could actually widen rather than reduce those inequalities, as it is the sections of the population who are initially healthier – specifically young, middle class males – who are the most likely to play.

During the past 20 years, although the gender gap in sports participation has narrowed (in conjunction with the upward trend in sport activity), age and social class differences have remained.[15]

'Bending the trend': improving physical activity levels

Because of the benefits of physical activity and the opportunities for improving physical activity levels, promotion of physical activity is one of the 'best buys' in public health available today.[16] With the established consensus on the benefits of moderate intensity physical activity, walking and cycling are clearly central to a strategy for promoting physical activity. Walking is the most natural of all physical activities, and cycling is a very accessible form of exercise. Both can form a central part of daily activity, and can be used for transport to and from work, for shopping and visiting friends.

Barriers to physical activity and sport

The main structural barriers or deterrents to walking and cycling are related to safety, attitudes, and unpleasant environment. They include:

– fear of traffic on roads, and broken pavements
– traffic fumes and pollution
– physical effort
– bad weather
– risk of bike theft, and
– public attitudes to cycling.[3]

Barriers to participation in sport include time and access to facilities. The cost of participation in sport has also become a deterrent for many, although cost more often appears to be a 'relative barrier', reducing the frequency of participation, rather than stopping people from participating at all.[17] In the six cities study, which looked at the provision of indoor sport facilities in Belfast, the London Borough of Camden, Cardiff, Chester, Glasgow and Liverpool, 40% of 16–24 year olds said the cost of playing was a barrier.[18]

Promotion of physical activity therefore needs to extend beyond the gymnasium and the badminton court to encompass activities that require a lower financial outlay, are accessible to more people, and promote greater levels of activity. The importance of walking and cycling becomes critical. Walking, for example, can lead to long-term health gain:[19] it can be of moderate intensity and can easily be done on most days of the week. Also, it can be performed alone or with other people, and it can be enjoyable and very convenient.

Transport and planning infrastructure

Fundamental to promoting physical activity are the development and implementation of health, transport and planning policies that encourage walking and cycling not just during leisure time, but as a means of daily travel. Such policies would facilitate a culture shift in favour of increased physical activity.[3] In areas where there are high concentrations of people living in poverty, addressing barriers such as safety and quality of the physical environment are important issues. However, while facilitation of healthier lifestyles is important, the solutions are not simple.

Promoting physical activity in many respects typifies the cross-sectoral approach to public health policy that is increasingly accepted as the way forward. Co-ordinated local action on transport and planning, within the context of an overarching and supportive national framework, involves the active collaboration of central and local government, the voluntary sector and business.

Sport and fitness facilities

The availability of fitness facilities will continue to be an important factor for promotion of physical activity, and can occur in conjunction with the development of wider health, transport and planning policies. If there is a supply of high-quality facilities accessible to the community, it is more likely that interests nurtured in childhood, whether in the home or in education, will be maintained in later life.[15]

A strategy of placing high-quality facilities in neighbourhoods has been implemented in inner Belfast, which makes a high and generous provision for indoor sport. Participation is extremely high, and the main reason for this is the level of provision. Belfast's facilities are sited within working class areas, and have lower user charges – factors which help make physical activity more accessible to lower socioeconomic groups.[18]

Children as a priority

Children should be a priority for promotion of physical activity. The needs of children from lower socioeconomic groups need particular attention in order to address the social gradient. Studies consistently point to low levels of physical activity among children and teenagers, and evidence suggests that children are less fit than they were 10 years ago.[3]

Physical activity is more likely to be continued in adulthood if it is established as a regular activity in childhood. Evidence from the six cities survey shows that the best predictor of whether individuals will remain regular sports participants throughout adulthood is not the volume of sport played at school, or the performance level achieved at that time, but the number of different sports to which individuals are introduced[15] (see Table 1).

Table 1   Sports socialisation and subsequent participation

Number of sports played when aged 16–19	Continuous (%)*	Interrupted (%)**
0	–	43
1	18	24
2	17	13
3	21	11
More	43	9

*   Played at least one sport regularly each year up to present age.
**   Played regularly in at least one, but not all years.
Source: See reference 15.

Children should be introduced to as many activities as possible while at school, and the sports curriculum should be enriched. The six cities research found that participation in sports in later life is most likely when young people acquire a broad set of sporting skills and interests, then continue to play regularly throughout the time when they leave full-time education, commence employment, change addresses and embark upon family formation. If young adults remain participants throughout these life events, the chances are that they will then continue to play throughout their 20s and 30s, and in many cases into their 40s and 50s.

Conclusion

Physical activity is desirable and should have a niche in health promotion. It should be promoted because it is enjoyable, not just because it is 'good for you'. Local and national planning and transport policies, including appropriate budget allocation, should encourage and enable walking and cycling as a part of daily life.

References

1   Powell KE, Thompson PD, Caspersen CJ, Kendrick JS. 1987. Physical activity and the incidence of coronary heart disease. *Annual Review of Public Health*; 8: 253–287.

2   Hardman A. Physical activity: how does it affect women's risk of CHD? In: Sharp I (ed.) 1994. *Coronary Heart Disease: Are Women Special?* London: National Forum for Coronary Heart Disease Prevention.

3   Sharp I. 1995. *Physical Activity: An Agenda for Action*. London: National Forum for Coronary Heart Disease Prevention.

4   Department of Health. 1995. *More People, More Active, More Often: Physical Activity in England. A Consultation Paper*. London: HMSO.

5   Health Education Authority and Sports Council. 1992. *Allied Dunbar National Fitness Survey: Main Findings*. London: Health Education Authority and Sports Council.

6   Hoinville E. 1995. Analysis of combined data from Allied Dunbar National Fitness Survey and HEANSAH (Health Education Authority National Survey of Activity and Health). Unpublished. Cited in: Health Education Authority. 1995. *Health Update 5: Physical Activity*. London: Health Education Authority.

7   Olszewska A, Roberts K. 1989. *Leisure and Lifestyle: A Comparative Analysis of Free Time*. London: Sage.

8   Cox B et al. 1993. *The Health and Lifestyle Survey: Seven Years On*. Aldershot: Dartmouth.

9   Health Education Authority. 1994. *Black and Minority Ethnic Groups in England*. London: Health Education Authority.

10 Cale L, Almond L. 1992. Physical activity levels of young children: a review of the evidence. *Health Education Journal*; 51: 94–99.

11 Cale L, Almond L. 1992. Physical activity levels of secondary aged children: a review. *Health Education Journal*; 51: 192–197.

12 Health Education Authority. 1991. *Tomorrow's Young Adults: 9–15 Year-olds Look at Alcohol, Drugs, Exercise and Smoking*. London: Health Education Authority. Cited in: Health Education Authority. 1995. *Health Update 5: Physical Activity*. London: Health Education Authority.

13 Roberts K. 1996. Young people, schools, sport and government policies. *Sport, Education and Society*; 1: 47–57.

14 Sports Council. 1988. *Sport in the Community: Into the 90s*. London: Sports Council.

15 Roberts K. 1993. *Sport and Health*. Liverpool: Department of Sociology, Social Policy and Social Work Studies. University of Liverpool. Unpublished.

16 Morris JN. 1994. Exercise in the prevention of coronary heart disease: today's best buy in public health. *Medicine and Science in Sports and Exercise*; 26: 807–814.

17 Coalter F. 1993. Sports participation: price or priorities? *Leisure Studies*; 12: 171–182.

18 Roberts K, Brodie DA. 1992. *Inner City Sport: Who Plays and What are the Benefits?* Culemborg (Netherlands): Giordano Bruno.

19 Hillsdon M, Thorogood M, Anstiss T, Morris J. 1995. Randomised control trials of physical activity promotion in free living populations: a review. *Journal of Epidemiology and Community Health*; 49: 448–455.

Chapter 10

Psychosocial factors in the workplace: their impact on coronary heart disease

Professor Tores Theorell

National Institute for Psychosocial Factors and Health, Stockholm

Introduction

Environmental factors have an important influence on health and on the risk of coronary heart disease. Within the workplace, environmental factors include not only the physical but also the psychosocial environment. Psychosocial aspects of work have an important influence over risk of coronary heart disease, and they can all be potentially modified. Three factors relevant to the work environment which have been the subject of research are:

- workload – the demands of work

- lack of control over an individual's own working conditions (low 'decision latitude'), including the possibility to influence decisions and learn new things

- social support, ie the degree to which an employee receives emotional and instrumental support from workmates and superiors at work, and from others outside work.

These factors often work in combination and have given rise to a theoretical model known as the 'demand–control–support' model.[1]

Other important factors include the influence of shift work[2] and the reward given in response to work undertaken.[3]

The psychosocial work environment and coronary risk

There are generally two ways to consider how the psychosocial work environment affects health. One is to consider individual susceptibility to stress in terms of the skills and abilities of the workforce. The other is to consider how an adverse working environment can generate stress.

These two factors act dynamically and are both potentially important. Individual stress management programmes for employees are more likely to have a lasting effect if there is concomitant effort to improve work organisation. Conversely, attention to work organisation will increase the motivation of employees to sustain the improved habits that they learn in individual stress management programmes.

One way to deal with stress is through individual counselling and stress management programmes. These can be of great potential benefit but this chapter focuses on the psychosocial conditions that could potentially be improved by means of work redesign.

There is increasing evidence to support the notion that aspects of work organisation in themselves contribute to the risk of coronary heart disease. Several studies have attempted to measure 'the aetiological fraction' associated with the psychosocial work environment – the proportion of coronary heart disease caused by poor psychosocial conditions at work.[1, 4]

A study in Stockholm, based on a large sample of patients with a first heart attack and age-matched healthy controls, suggested that 11% of the risk of a first heart attack among working men below the age of 55 could be attributed to a combination of high psychological demands and lack of control (or low 'decision latitude') at work.[5] The corresponding fraction for women was slightly higher at 13%. These findings were true after controlling for age, biomedical risk factors, social class, and chest pain preceding the heart attack. Other research suggests that, if these factors are combined with a shift work schedule, the 'aetiological fraction' exceeds 25%.[4] It is clear that the 'aetiological fraction' depends on how terms are defined and on the methods used for measuring both work demands and control over working conditions. But despite these difficulties the calculations of 'aetiological fraction' have had similar results in different studies.

There is a strikingly consistent association between measurements of poor psychosocial work environment and risk of coronary heart disease. Of the many studies which have examined this association, the vast majority have shown a positive link. When an objective evaluation of psychosocial working conditions is used, poor working conditions may increase the relative risk of coronary heart disease by between 20% and 100%.[5, 6] When people are asked to make their own assessment of their psychosocial working conditions, the relative risk increases by a factor of between two and four.

The Whitehall study of British civil servants[7], based on a large cohort study, found that those who described a low decision latitude on two occasions, three years apart, had a relative risk of developing coronary heart disease during follow-up of 1.9 compared to other participants. The relationship was significant both for men and women and held even after adjustment for negative affectivity (a psychological tendency to describe everything in life in negative terms), social class and all the accepted biomedical risk factors. In this study, psychological 'demand' made no difference. (For more information on the Whitehall study, see Chapter 2.)

'Job strain' – a combination of lack of control and high psychological demands – has, however, been associated in many studies with an increased risk of heart attack. For example, in a large study carried out in Sweden, several thousand men who had had a first heart attack were compared to controls from the general population.[8] The men were grouped by means of an indirect measurement system, based on the general working population in Sweden, according to their level of 'job strain'. Those who had had a heart attack were more likely to have suffered from 'job strain'.

In the same study, lack of influence over planning work content and working hours were also associated with an increased risk of heart attack.[8] The combinations that carried the highest risk were: a hectic work schedule and lack of influence over working hours; and a hectic work schedule and lack of influence over planning. Each of these combinations was associated with a relative risk of 1.6.

Smoking has been considered to be a possible avenue for the association between working conditions and coronary heart disease risk – ie people smoke more when job conditions are poor. In some studies smoking has been associated with 'job strain'. Smokers who are experiencing 'job strain' find it more difficult to give up smoking, and are less likely to quit.[1, 9]

Which factors are important?

The psychosocial work environment seems to be consistently associated with an increased risk of coronary heart disease, but the different elements need to be considered independently. The original demand-control model, introduced by Karasek in 1979, included work demands (equivalent to 'stress') and lack of control (or lack of 'decision latitude'). More recently, social support has been included in the model.

Thus the three main risk factors in the psychosocial work environment are: control over work, work 'demand', and social support.

Of these, the most important factor seems to be control over work, which has the most consistent relationship with risk of coronary heart disease. A lower level of control is associated with an increased risk of coronary heart disease. This may be exacerbated by work demands; when people have less control over their work, then higher demands may increase their risk.[1]

Epidemiological studies have shown that between 30% and 40% of the variance in coronary heart disease mortality and/or morbidity risk between different occupations can be explained by the control factor, whereas only 7% has been explained by the 'demand' factor.[1] The proportion of the variance in coronary heart disease risk attributable to 'control' seems to add to that which can be attributed to income differences.

The worst combination appears to be low social support combined with a low level of control and high demand, a combination known as 'iso-strain'. A study based on self-reported working conditions in Swedish men who were followed up for eight years, showed that the 20% of men with 'iso-strain' died eight years earlier from cardiovascular disease than those 20% with the best combination.[10]

The amount of reward given for work effort has also been shown to be indirectly associated with an increased risk of coronary heart disease. A study of blue-collar workers found that those who perceived that they were given low rewards for their effort had an increased risk of coronary heart disease.[3] This may be a potential area for action. Rewards could be financial, or could be based on ways of promoting self-esteem or ways of enhancing an individual's capacity to assert control over his or her total life situation.

Both the reward-effort model and the demand-control-support models have been shown to supplement each other in predicting coronary heart disease. Lack of control and unfavourable reward-effort imbalance both contribute independently of one another and of other risk factors such as the biomedical risk factors and social class.[11]

Lack of control at work

A study of men aged 45–54 years of age, over a 10-year period, found that working men who had had a first heart attack had experienced a greater lack of control at work than other working men.[12] Even after adjusting for chest pain preceding the heart attack, social class and accepted biomedical risk factors, those men who had experienced least control over their work (ie those in the bottom quartile) had a relative risk of 1.9 of developing a first myocardial infarction. This therefore suggests that interventions in terms of the nature of the job or task and providing other means of support, may help prevent heart attacks.

Bus driving has been identified as an occupation with high 'job-strain'. In the two largest cities in Sweden, bus drivers have a relative risk of coronary heart disease of between 1.5 and 1.6, whereas there is no increased risk in other cities. This suggests a combined effect of environmental risk factors. Some of the increased risk is due to the well known risk factors such as sedentary work and smoking. However, there are also psychosocial factors such as accumulated lack of control that the bus drivers have in stressful situations.[13] Practical solutions such as introducing bus lanes have been tested in Sweden and found to greatly reduce tensions for the bus drivers, although other drivers also have to be educated. This is a complex task which involves society as a whole, but which needs to be undertaken if job strain is to be reduced.

Does the psychosocial work environment explain social class inequalities in coronary heart disease?

The extent to which social class inequalities in coronary heart disease can be explained by differences in the psychosocial work environment is not yet known.

It is possible that the relationship between lack of control at work and increased risk of coronary heart disease simply reflects the relationship between social class and coronary heart disease risk – ie those in lower social classes tend to have a lower level of control at work. However, several studies have shown that the association remains, even after controlling for social class.[1, 4, 6]

However, the same is not true for work 'demand'. This tends to increase further up the social scale, while risk of coronary heart disease falls. This suggests that it is control rather than demand that has most bearing on the differences in coronary heart disease risk between different occupational groups.

How does job strain affect coronary heart disease risk?

There is some debate about the mechanisms by which the psychosocial work environment may affect the risk of coronary heart disease.[1, 5]

The relationship may be mediated by psychophysiological changes. One of these may be elevated blood pressure. However, studies have not found a consistent association between job strain and conventional blood pressure measurements.[5, 6] Nevertheless, most studies of repeated fully automated measures of variations in blood pressure during everyday activities have shown a relationship between job strain and blood pressure during working hours. These could be due to the action of the sympathetic adrenal system.[5, 6]

What can be done?

The evidence suggests that the most important factors to address are lack of control over work and low levels of social support. Lack of control can be addressed, for example, by designing job rotation schemes, or by giving employees more authority over decisions which affect their working conditions. Holding regular staff meetings, where employees can raise important issues, can help increase employees' sense of control.

Several studies have indicated a relationship between shift work and risk of coronary heart disease.[2, 4, 14] Shift work is a strain on an organism since adaptation is slow and therefore the body does not receive sufficient sleep during aroused day hours and has to be aroused at night when the biological systems are ill-adapted. The end result is a chronic state of arousal which may explain susceptibility to coronary heart disease. Shift work may also encourage lifestyles which increase arousal, such as smoking and certain dietary habits.

Shifts could be organised to accommodate natural biological rhythms in a better way. Several experiments are underway in Sweden which show promising results.[14]

Other studies have shown that organisational change can bring about an endocrinological response in employees and that cortisol levels are reduced when the work situation improves. It seems to be important to prepare employees for organisational change.[15] A recent study in Sweden has shown that a combined approach including individual counselling and better work organisation resulting in improved support and decision latitude for the employees may result in improved (less atherogenic) lipoprotein patterns. Such a change was not observed in the control group and it could not be explained by changes in diet or other changes in life habits.[16]

Conclusion

A sense of control over a person's working life is an important factor in the relationship between the working environment and the risk of coronary heart disease, and it is a factor which can be altered. When the psychosocial work environment improves – for example by increasing the number of staff meetings, giving increased attention to support and control for the employees in the organisation – the individual's sense of control improves, and this in turn affects the person's physiology in ways which could significantly reduce his or her risk of coronary heart disease. Targeting and improving the psychosocial work environment is therefore an important part of the effort to reduce coronary heart disease.

References

1   Karasek RA, Theorell T. 1990. *Healthy Work: Stress, Productivity, and the Reconstruction of Working Life*. New York: Basic Books.

2   Knutsson A. 1989. Shift work and coronary heart disease. *Scandinavian Journal of Social Medicine*; suppl. 44.

3   Siegrist J, Peter R, Junge A, Cremer P, Seidel D. 1990. Low status control, high effort at work and ischemic heart disease: Prospective evidence from blue-collar men. *Social Science and Medicine*; 10: 1127–1134.

4   Kristensen TS, 1995. The demand-control-support model: Methodological challenges for future research. *Stress Medicine*; 11: 17–26.

5   Theorell T, Karasek RA. 1996. Current issues relating to psychosocial job strain and cardiovascular disease research. *Journal of Occupational Health Psychology*; 1: 9–26.

6   Schnall P L, Landsbergis PA. 1994. Job strain and cardiovascular disease. *Annual Review of Public Health*; 15: 381–411.

7   Bosma H, Marmot MG, Hemingway H, Nicholson AC, Brunner E, Stansfeld SA. 1997. Low job control and risks of coronary heart disease in Whitehall II (prospective cohort study). *British Medical Journal*; 314: 558–565.

8   Hammar N, Alfredsson L, Theorell T. 1994. Job characteristics and the incidence of myocardial infarction. *International Journal of Epidemiology*; 23: 277–284.

9   Green KL, Johnson JV. 1990. The effects of psychosocial work organization on patterns of cigarette smoking among male chemical plant employees. *American Journal of Public Health*; 80: 1368–1371.

10   Johnson JV, Hall EM, Theorell T. 1989. Combined effects of job strain and social isolation on cardiovascular disease morbidity and mortality in a random sample of the Swedish male working population. *Scandinavian Journal of Work Environment and Health*; 15: 271–279.

11   Bosma H, Peter R, Siegrist J, Marmot M. 1998. Two alternative job stress models and the risk of coronary heart disease. *American Journal of Public Health*; 88 (1): 68–74.

12   Theorell T, Tsutsumi A, Hallquist J, Reutervall C, Fredlund P, Hogstedt C, Emlund N, Johnson J and the Stockholm Heart Epidemiology Program (SHEEP). 1998. Decision latitude, job strain and myocardial infarction: A study of working men in Stockholm. *American Journal of Public Health*; 88 (3): 382–388.

13   Emdad R, Belkic K, Theorell T, Wennberg A, Hagman M, Johansson L, Savic C, Cizinsky S. 1996. Electrocortical responses to ecologically relevant visual stimuli among professional drivers with and without cardiovascular disease. *Integrative Physiological and Behavioral Science*; 31 (2): 96–111.

14   Lennernäs MA-C. 1993. *Nutrition and Shift Work*. Academic thesis. Stockholm (Sweden): Karolinska Institute.

15   Theorell T, Ort-Gomér K, Moser V, Undén A–L, Eriksson I. 1995. Endocrine markers during job intervention. *Work and Stress*; 9 (1): 67–76.

16   Orth-Gomér K, Eriksson I, Moser V, Theorell T, Fredlund P. 1994. Lipid lowering through work stress reduction. *International Journal of Behavioural Medicine*; 1 (3): 204–214.

Chapter 11

Healthy work: policy and action

Professor Tom Cox and Dr Amanda Griffiths

Centre for Organisational Health and Development, Department of Psychology, University of Nottingham

Introduction

In the UK, 745 million working days are lost each year due to sickness and invalidity.[1] Of these, 65 million (9%) are caused by coronary heart disease. The comparable figures for cardiovascular disease (which includes coronary heart disease and stroke) are 123 million working days, representing 17% of the total. Working days lost due to coronary heart disease morbidity are estimated to cost British industry £4,800 million a year in lost production.[2] The lost production costs due to deaths from coronary heart disease are estimated at an additional £1,600 million a year.

This chapter considers the concept of healthy work, and the formulation of national and organisational policies for healthy work, including cardiovascular health. It focuses on the general usefulness of a problem-solving approach to hazard reduction and health promotion. It recognises the need to consider carefully national differences within Europe when formulating policy and planning action for healthy work and cardiovascular health.

What is healthy work?

Current UK and European Union (EU) health and safety legislation places duties on employers to ensure that work is 'safe and without risk to health'. While the concept of 'safe work' appears relatively straightforward and has a long history, the concept of 'healthy work' is both more complex and more recent.

The most common perception of what constitutes 'healthy work' is that which is without risk to physical health. However, this definition is inadequate in several ways. Firstly, the concept of 'healthy work' goes beyond that which is without risk to health, and logically includes consideration of the health-positive aspects of work (aspects of work which are beneficial to health). Secondly, it must make reference to the psychological and social aspects of health as well as to the physical aspects. 'Healthy work' is work that does not threaten but which maintains and enhances the physical, psychological and social health of the worker.

Threats to cardiovascular health arise both from aspects of people's work and from their non-work lives and social living conditions. The concept of 'healthy work' is important not only to our understanding and management of the impact of work on cardiovascular health, but is also important in relation to the interactions which occur between work, non-work life and social living conditions.

The threat to cardiovascular health through work is not only through exposure to the more tangible hazards of the workplace, such as tobacco smoke, but also as a result of exposure to the psychosocial and organisational hazards of work. These reflect the design and management of work and work systems, and of the organisations in which they exist.[3]

Knowing what constitutes healthy work and what threatens or promotes cardiovascular health at work is necessary but not sufficient in itself for effective management of this issue. It is necessary to have:
– complementary scientific and legal frameworks
– a supporting policy, and
– practical strategies.

The effective development of healthy work, including cardiovascular health, involves not only traditional workplace health promotion but also hazard reduction. The latter must consider not just the more tangible hazards of work but also the psychosocial and organisational hazards.

The role of policy is, in part, to translate the intellectual and legal frameworks into a practical strategy, and, in part, to facilitate that strategy. The intellectual framework is provided by research reviewed in Chapter 10 of this report. One possible legal framework is briefly discussed below.

A legal framework

One legal framework for healthy work is provided, in part, by the current UK and EU legislation in the area of health and safety.[4-6] For example, the Health and Safety at Work Act 1974 places a duty on the employer "to provide and maintain a safe working environment which is, so far as is reasonably practicable, safe, without risks to health and adequate as regards facilities and arrangements for their welfare at work". The 1992 Management of Health and Safety at Work Regulations place a responsibility on employers to assess the health risks at work and to put in place procedures and mechanisms to prevent or reduce those risks. The 1992 workplace regulations also state that provision must be made to protect non-smokers from the discomfort caused by tobacco smoke in rest rooms or rest areas. This legal framework has provided a spur to thinking about the need for and nature of hazard reduction at work. A recurrent theme in this legislation has been the need to adopt a systematic, problem-solving approach to work-related health problems and hazard reduction.

Employers therefore have a duty to assess all work-related risks to the safety and health of their employees, and where necessary take reasonable actions to reduce those risks. It is made clear that the notion of all risks includes those associated with the design and management of work (psychosocial and organisational hazards). While usable risk assessment and risk reduction techniques have been developed and tested for the more tangible hazards of work, their application to the psychosocial and organisational hazards is only now being explored.

Generic risk assessment and risk reduction strategies are described in many different health and safety regulations, codes of practice and guidance notes published in both the UK and the EU. An early example is provided by the UK Control of Substances Hazardous to Health Regulations 1988,[7] and the subsequent amendment 1990.[8] These regulations obliged employers to undertake an assessment of health risk to employees for activities associated with substances hazardous to health and, in parallel, to assess the effectiveness of existing control systems. The essence of these regulations was to ensure a proactive approach to assessment and prevention or control of exposure.

The approach was set out in six steps which together describe the typical cycle of control for risk assessment and risk reduction:

1 Identification of hazards

2 Assessment of associated risk

3 Design and implementation of appropriate control strategies with an emphasis on risk reduction

4 Monitoring of effectiveness of control strategies

5 Re-assessment of risk

6 Review of information and training needs of employees exposed to hazards.

This cycle of actions has been termed the 'control cycle'. It has been shown to be effective in relation to the more tangible hazards of work, and is being adapted for use with psychosocial and organisational hazards. Its use should aid the development of healthy work by reducing risks to health. What is required for cardiovascular health is an 'appropriate and adequate' assessment procedure and a reasonable hazard reduction programme where this is indicated from the available evidence. The control cycle applied to cardiovascular health has to be 'good enough' to identify and reduce any major risks and to take out the worst case scenarios. Employers have a general duty in health and safety law to carry out risk assessments and enact hazard reduction where necessary.

Employers have no statutory duty to support health promotion activities in the workplace unless, of course, such activities are clearly indicated as an appropriate and reasonable response to an important health risk. However, traditional health promotion activities may provide a useful adjunct to hazard reduction in relation to coronary heart disease. Furthermore, the activities necessary to establish the need for and planning of such programmes can be easily incorporated in the assessment phase of the control cycle.

Monitoring and evaluation

Monitoring and evaluation are essential for the development of effective hazard reduction and effective health promotion. Performance should be measured and evaluated against predetermined plans and any relevant standards or targets, considering not only the outcomes but also the process involved in implementing those plans and the compliance with standards and targets.

Standards and targets for cardiovascular health can represent what is ideally possible and desirable, or what is tolerable or practicable in a given work situation. Much of the UK and EU legislation on health and safety, particularly in relation to inspection and enforcement, sets out minimum standards: what is tolerable or judged practicable in a given situation. Other organisations and agencies, such as research bodies, may provide insights into standards of excellence and set higher targets: what is desirable. Continuous improvement of health in the workplace should be set against this model, ever striving to close the gap between the two.

What can be done?

Legislation could be used to prescribe a comprehensive and detailed system of workplace control for cardiovascular health to ensure minimal exposure to hazards and to regulate workers' behaviour in a safe and healthy way. Or it could set out general principles for the design and management of work and work systems, and for behaviour at work, and provide guidance on the application of those principles. Current UK and EU legislation adopts the later strategy, partly because there is not yet sufficient scientific evidence to support the comprehensive and detailed prescription which the first strategy demands for cardiovascular health. In any case, it is not clear whether legislative control, on its own, is an effective method of changing the work behaviour of individuals or of their organisations.

The alternative or complementary approach to legislation is to formulate general principles of healthy work and cardiovascular health and procedures for hazard reduction and for health promotion, and to provide training and other guidance on their application. To be effective, such an approach would require the publication of clear policies on healthy work and cardiovascular health at both national and organisational levels. This might be best achieved within the framework provided by existing health and safety regulations and related guidance, and incorporated within existing policy statements on health and safety.

A prescription for a good policy

An effective policy in this area must arguably integrate the intellectual and legal frameworks supporting the development of healthy work with a strategy for hazard reduction and health promotion. It must encourage, legitimise and resource associated actions. A natural vehicle for such a policy, at an organisational level, would be the company's existing health and safety policy. This might be usefully developed through a policy document on healthy work, which would impact on cardiovascular health as well as protecting against other health risks. A good policy document, in this area, should include:

- A concise statement of the objectives of the policy and, in this case, a clear vision of healthy work for cardiovascular health

- A commitment to healthy work backed by intellectual and legal argument

- An account of the costs and benefits of action and inaction with respect to healthy work and cardiovascular health

- A statement of achievable standards. This could also include statements of minimum acceptable standards and standards of excellence set against realistic timescales.

- Guidance on relevant hazard reduction and health promotion techniques with examples of good practice

- Details of organisational arrangements and resources to support action to achieve certain standards. Action must include general education.

- Guidance on evaluation of actions.

Elements of such a policy document could be developed and published at a national level both to provide a possible outline for organisational policies and to encourage the formulation of those policies. Any governmental policy could usefully focus on the legitimisation of concern for cardiovascular health at work, its status as a health and safety issue, the provision of guidance on good practice in the process of risk assessment and risk reduction, workplace health promotion, the education of managers, trades union representatives and other employees, and the training of government advisers and inspectors.

National and international policies

Significant differences between European countries must be taken into account in the formulation of any European policy on healthy work and cardiovascular health. Such differences have been noted in the literature and are of scientific importance. They concern not only linguistic and cultural differences but also differences in constitutional thinking and practice. While it is useful to reach broad agreement at a European level, given these differences it might not be sensible to standardise all aspects of any policy or associated programme on healthy work and cardiovascular health across countries. It is important to take into account the local context, and to tailor policies and associated programmes of hazard reduction and health promotion accordingly. Agreement on a general framework might be best achieved at European level but detailed policy and programme formulation as described above should be developed at a national and organisational level.

References

1   British Heart Foundation. 1997. *Coronary Heart Disease Statistics: 1997 Edition*. London: British Heart Foundation.

2   Maniadikis N, Rayner M. 1998. *Coronary Heart Disease Statistics: Economic Costs Supplement*. London: British Heart Foundation.

3   Cox T. 1993. *Stress Research and Stress Management*. Sudbury: HSE Books.

4   *Health and Safety at Work Act, 1974*. London: HMSO.

5   *Management of Health and Safety at Work Regulations, 1992*. London: HMSO.

6   *EC Framework Directive 89/391/EEC*.

7   *Control of Substances Hazardous to Health Regulations, 1988*. London: HMSO.

8   *Control of Substances Hazardous to Health (Amendment) Regulations, 1990. Statutory instrument no: 2026*. London: HMSO.

Chapter 12

The impact of health care on inequalities in coronary heart disease

Professor Rod Griffiths

NHS Executive West Midlands Regional Office

Introduction

What can be done to reduce the social variations in coronary heart disease? What should be done? Should the focus be on health services, access to health care, or lifestyle? Can the different issues be disentangled? There are three confounding factors: different service levels in different districts, historic patterns of access to health care, and significant areas of deprivation.

The West Midlands Regional Health Authority has been concerned for some time about how deprivation and access to health care can influence health. This chapter focuses on the relationship between deprivation and coronary heart disease, using routine information available to the NHS Executive West Midlands, including mortality data from the Office for National Statistics, West Midlands hospital admissions statistics, and 1991 census data. The region has a population of 5.2 million: half rural, half urban. There are significant numbers of ethnic minorities and higher than average rates of coronary heart disease. Within the region, there are 400,000 people who are in the most deprived 10% of the national census sample. The areas these people live in are both concentrated and isolated areas of deprivation.

Deprivation and coronary heart disease mortality

There is a clear and significant relationship between deprivation and the likelihood of dying of coronary heart disease among under-75 year old men: those in the more deprived groups are more likely to die of the disease (see Figure 1). Those in the highest band of deprivation have a standardised mortality about 70% higher than those in the lowest band. However, this trend disappears for those aged 75 and over. The position in women is different, with no trend in standardised mortality ratios for coronary heart disease across the deprivation groups (see Figure 2).

Figure 1 *Deprivation and deaths from coronary heart disease, directly standardised rates, men, West Midlands, 1994/95–1996/97**

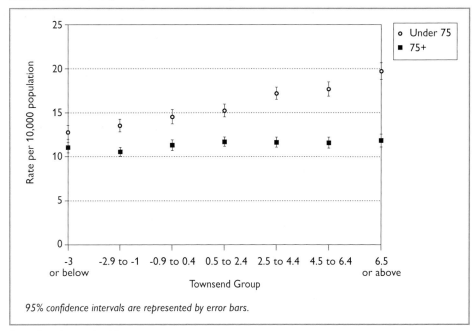

95% confidence intervals are represented by error bars.

Source: See references 1 and 2.

Figure 2 *Deprivation and deaths from coronary heart disease, directly standardised rates, women, West Midlands, 1994/95–1996/97**

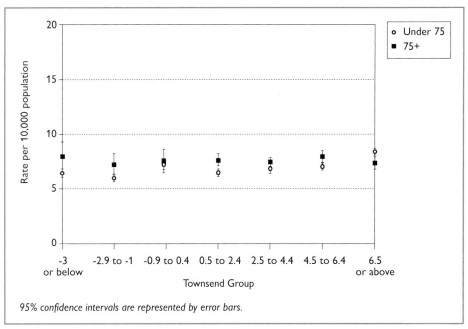

95% confidence intervals are represented by error bars.

Source: See references 1 and 2.

There is also a relationship between deprivation* and mortality for all the major disease groups except for breast cancer and skin cancer for which the trend, as expected, is in the opposite direction.

---

*   In these data, deprivation is measured by the Townsend Score which remains reasonably stable between different census years. The data are based on enumeration districts taken from postcodes on mortality and hospital admission records, as these bear more relation to general practice and can be mapped by deprivation score. Ward and constituency boundaries are arbitrary: they are designed to produce constituencies of a particular size and bear no relation to the organisation of health care. District boundaries have similar arbitrary elements and since the recent rash of mergers are often so big that social variation is lost within the boundary.

Deprivation and hospital admissions for coronary heart disease

There is also a clear and significant relationship between deprivation and the hospital episode rate for coronary heart disease (the number of admissions to hospital per 100,000 population). It is well established that those in more deprived groups are more likely to be admitted to hospital.[3]

What causes these trends? Are they caused by health services? Are poor people treated badly in hospital? Do they not explain their symptoms properly? Is it to do with getting them to hospital? Or is the trend caused by something that happens before then? One way to find the answer is to look at the relationship between deprivation and the coronary heart disease case fatality rate.

Deprivation and coronary heart disease case fatality

The coronary heart disease case fatality rate is the proportion of hospital admissions for coronary heart disease which end in death. It might be expected that there could be a number of reasons why poorer people might be less likely to survive. It is possible that they have additional causes of ill health, that they have poorer nutrition, or are less adept at making their symptoms clear. In fact there is no trend in either men or women.

It is quite clear that, once a person is admitted to hospital with coronary heart disease, their chances of survival are not dependent on where they have come from. (See Figures 3 and 4. These graphs are based on aggregation of several years' data across the whole of the West Midlands and are therefore based on very large numbers of admissions. The statistical confidence intervals are narrow and the conclusions therefore fairly reliable.)

Figure 3 *Deprivation and case fatality for coronary heart disease deaths, men, West Midlands 1994/95–1996/97*

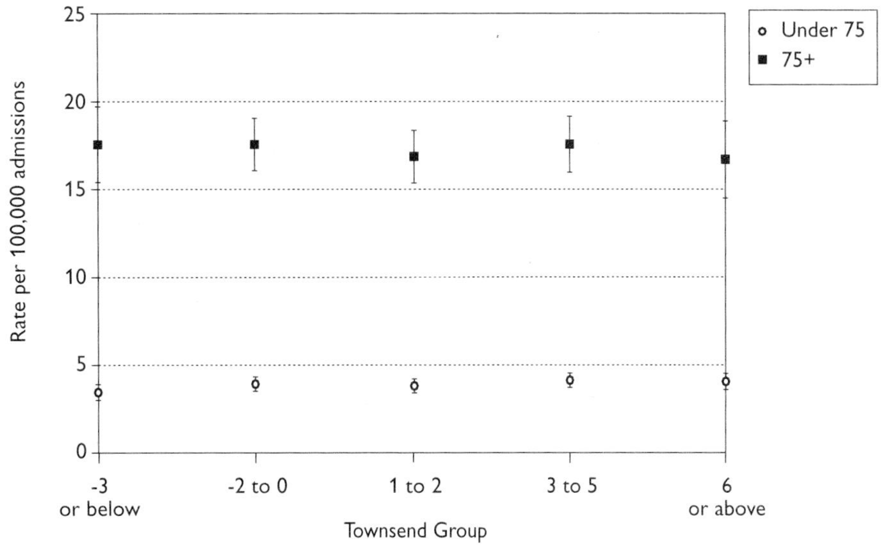

95% confidence intervals are represented by error bars.

Source: See references 2 and 4.

Figure 4 *Deprivation and case fatality for coronary heart disease deaths, women, West Midlands 1994/95–1996/97*

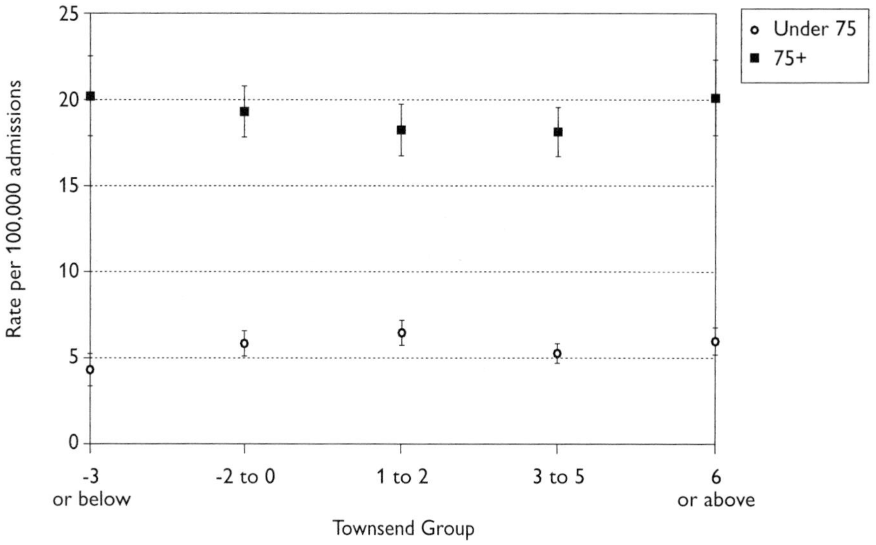

95% confidence intervals are represented by error bars.

Source: See references 2 and 4.

Conclusions

It is quite clear that males under the age of 75 from poorer communities are more likely to die of heart disease than those from better off communities. They are also more likely to be admitted to hospital. Once they get to hospital the chances of survival are the same for everyone. The implication is quite clear. The causes of the extra deaths must act outside hospital.

Other analyses have examined the proportions of cases from the different communities who die at home, on the way to hospital and in hospital. Once again there is little difference between the groups, and such differences that do exist are far too small to account for the difference in mortality.

This suggests that a strategy to reduce the excess burden of coronary heart disease mortality associated with poverty needs to consider a much more fundamental look at the possible causes rather than treatment, and needs to find ways of mobilising social effort to combat them.

Options for action

Health promotion

The chance of successfully reducing the social inequalities in health can be increased if districts set local targets which are challenging but sensible. It is remarkable how little is spent on health promotion and how little attention has been directed to developing the evidence base, when one considers the magnitude of the health problems that need to be addressed.

Smoking is the biggest single health hazard, and the largest single preventable cause of coronary heart disease. The issue of action on smoking should be raised with district managers at each district review. It does not appear that huge amounts of money need to be spent to spur significant activity. However, the problem with health promotion – including action on smoking – is that it takes a long time to have an impact on statistics, even if local initiatives are successful.

Improving quality of care in hospitals

As there are between 30% and 40% more admissions to hospital from deprived areas, there is a need to target improvements in hospital care to some degree at deprived groups and this need possibly justifies the excessive attention that has been paid to the resource allocation formula. Since half of the deaths from coronary heart disease take place in hospital, improving death rates in hospitals could have an immediate impact on national targets for coronary heart disease although it will only impact on poverty to the extent that poor people are more likely to be admitted.

In the West Midlands, a continuous region-wide audit of thrombolytic therapy has been undertaken. Data have been fed back to trusts and health authorities. This has led to a continuous improvement in 'pain to needle' and 'door to needle' times. A number of hospitals have shown that they can sustain door to needle times of about 30 minutes while others still have difficulties in breaking an hour on a regular basis. It has been shown that the time from call to GP and arrival at hospital can be halved by the GP dialling 999 immediately on receipt of a suggestive history. Call to door times of 30 minutes can be achieved by this means on a regular basis. The most difficult delay to tackle is that between onset of symptoms and call to the GP. So far, efforts have concentrated on getting the GP and hospital delays down to acceptable limits, eg 30 minutes each. A further attack on pain to call times is being delayed until it is clear that the NHS can cope well with patients once they arrive at hospital.

Changes such as those described above do save lives but it is clear that they cannot remove the social gradient in coronary heart disease. Much more action is required outside hospital and it would be wrong for too much attention to be wasted on advances in secondary care that will always be dealing with the problem late in the day.

References

1   Office for National Statistics. Mortality data for 1994–1997.

2   Office of Population Censuses and Surveys. 1991 Census.

3   Griffiths R (ed). 1992. *Report of the Regional Director of Public Health*. Birmingham: West Midlands Regional Health Authority.

4   NHS Executive West Midlands Regional Information System.

List of participants

The following people participated in the National Heart Forum expert meeting on Social Variations in Coronary Heart Disease: Possibilities for Action, from which this report derives.

Dr Jane Ashwell, Department of Health

Dr Madhavi Bajekal, Department of General Practice, St Mary's Hospital Medical School, London

Dr Deborah Baker, School of Social Sciences, University of Bath

Dr Mel Bartley, Nuffield College, Oxford

Ms Hilary Beach, Health Promotion Wales

Ms Michaela Benzeval, King's Fund Institute

Dr H Binysh, The Royal Institute of Public Health and Hygiene

Dr Kathy Binysh, Department of Health

Sir Douglas Black

Dr David Blane, Department of Psychiatry, Charing Cross and Westminster Medical School, London

Ms Isobel Bowler, Health Education Authority

Dr Eric Brunner, Department of Epidemiology and Public Health, University College London Medical School

Ms Lisa Bullard-Cawthorne, Medical Education Development Officer, National Heart Forum

Ms Mary Cayzer, Community Practitioners' and Health Visitors' Association (formerly the Health Visitors' Association)

Dr John Coope, Anticipatory Care Teams

Professor Tom Cox, Centre for Organisational Health and Development, Department of Psychology, University of Nottingham

Mr Ray Cross, Department of Health

Professor George Davey Smith, Department of Social Medicine, University of Bristol

Ms Elizabeth Dowler, Centre for Human Nutrition, London School of Hygiene and Tropical Medicine

Ms Maria Duggan, Institute for Public Policy Research

Dr Jonathan Elford, University Department of Public Health, Royal Free Hospital School of Medicine, London

Ms Kathy Elliott, Health Education Authority

Ms Haroulla Filakti, Office of Population Censuses and Surveys

Professor Hilary Graham, Department of Applied Social Studies, University of Warwick

Mr Phelim M Green, Department of Health and Social Services, Northern Ireland

Professor Rod Griffiths, NHS Executive West Midlands Regional Office

Ms Hilary Groom, British Nutrition Foundation

Professor Dr Louise Gunning-Schepers, Institute for Social Medicine, Academic Medical Centre, Amsterdam

Dr Philip Hannaford, ICRF Clinical Research Fellow and Royal College of General Practitioners

Mr A Hedley Brown, Society of Cardiothoracic Surgeons

Mr Ken Judge, King's Fund Institute

Professor Desmond Julian, Chairman, National Heart Forum

Dr Rajendra Kale, British Medical Journal

Dr Diana Kuh, Department of Epidemiology and Public Health, University College London Medical School

Ms Henrietta Lang, Health policy consultant

Dr Tim Lang, Institute of Food Policy, Thames Valley University, London

Ms Suzi Leather, Food policy consultant

Dr Andrew Lyon, Forward Scotland (formerly Coordinator of the Glasgow Healthy City Project)

Professor Michael Marmot, International Centre for Health and Society, Department of Epidemiology and Public Health, University College London

Dr Alan Marsh, Policy Studies Institute

Dr Alan Maryon Davis, Faculty of Public Health Medicine

Ms Valerie Mason, British Heart Foundation

Dr Hamish McInnes, Sports Council

Professor Klim McPherson, Health Promotion Sciences Unit, London School of Hygiene and Tropical Medicine

Dr HRP Meldrum, British Medical Association

Professor Jerry Morris, London School of Hygiene and Tropical Medicine

Dr Noel Olsen, Director of Public Health, Plymouth Health Authority

Dr Luise Parsons, East London and the City Health Authority

Professor Brian Pentecost, British Heart Foundation

Mr David Pollock, Action on Smoking and Health (ASH)

Dr Chris Power, Department of Epidemiology and Biostatistics, Institute of Child Health, London

Mr Geof Rayner, Public Health Alliance

Dr Mike Rayner, Department of Public Health and Primary Care, Oxford University

Lord Rea, Parliamentary Food and Health Forum, and individual member of the National Heart Forum

Dr Rudolph A Riemersma, Royal College of Physicians of Edinburgh

Professor Ken Roberts, Department of Sociology, Social Policy and Social Work Studies, University of Liverpool

Ms Julia Robinson, The Coronary Prevention Group

Dr Lesley A Rogers, Assistant Director, National Heart Forum

Dr Nicola Royan, Society of Occupational Medicine

Ms Maggie Sanderson, British Dietetic Association

Professor AG Shaper, Vice Chair, National Heart Forum

Ms Imogen Sharp, Director, National Heart Forum

Ms Olivia Simmonds, Association of Primary Care Facilitators

Dr Rosalind Skinner, The Scottish Office, Home and Health Department

Professor Tores Theorell, National Institute for Psychosocial Factors and Health, Stockholm

Dr Michael Turner, Family Heart Association

Ms Sally Turner, British Association for Cardiac Rehabilitation

Ms Sarah Veale, Trades Union Congress

Dr Goya Wannamethee, Department of Public Health, Royal Free Hospital School of Medicine, London

Ms Patricia Ward, Consumers' Association

Dr Virginia Warren, Faculty of Public Health Medicine

Mr Mark Weston, Leeds Health Promotion Service

Ms Margaret Whitehead, Independent consultant

Professor Richard Wilkinson, Trafford Centre for Medical Research, University of Sussex

Ms Pauline Willie, British Heart Foundation

Ms Lynn Young, Royal College of Nursing

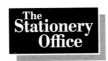

Published by The Stationery Office and available from:

The Publications Centre
(mail, telephone and fax orders only)
PO Box 276, London SW8 5DT
General enquiries 0171 873 0011
Telephone orders 0171 873 9090
Fax orders 0171 873 8200

The Stationery Office Bookshops
123 Kingsway, London WC2B 6PQ
0171 242 6393 Fax 0171 242 6394
68–69 Bull Street, Birmingham B4 6AD
0121 236 9696   Fax 0121 236 9699
33 Wine Street, Bristol BS1 2BQ
0117 9264306 Fax 0117 9294515
9–21 Princess Street, Manchester M60 8AS
0161 834 7201 Fax 0161 833 0634
16 Arthur Street, Belfast BT1 4GD
01232 238451 Fax 01232 235401
The Stationery Office Oriel Bookshop
The Friary, Cardiff CF1 4AA
01222 395548 Fax 01222 384347
71 Lothian Road, Edinburgh EH3 9AZ
0131 228 4181   Fax 0131 622 7017

The Stationery Office's Accredited Agents
(see Yellow Pages)

and through good booksellers